FUEL
YOUR BODY

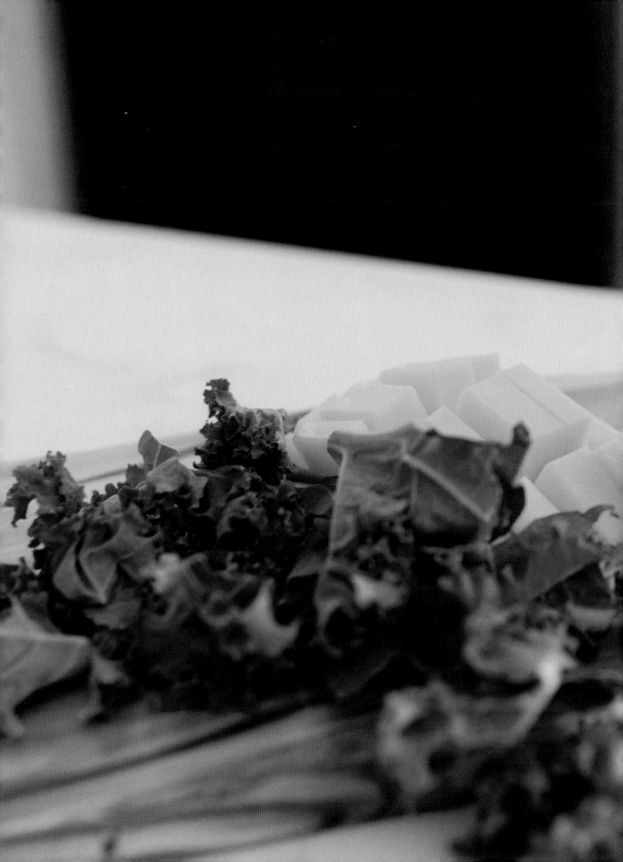

# FUEL
## YOUR BODY

*HOW TO COOK AND EAT FOR PEAK PERFORMANCE*

**ANGIE ASCHE**, MS, RD, CSSD

*FOUNDER OF ELEAT SPORTS NUTRITION*

A SURREY BOOK

## AGATE

CHICAGO

Printed in China

Library of Congress Cataloging-in-Publication Data
Names: Asche, Angie, author.
Title: Fuel your body : how to cook and eat for peak performance: 77
    simple, nutritious, whole-food recipes for every athlete / Angie Asche,
    MS, RD, CSSD Founder of Eleat Sports Nutrition.
Description: Chicago : Agate Publishing, 2021. | Includes index.
Identifiers: LCCN 2020040118 (print) | LCCN 2020040119
(ebook) | ISBN
    9781572842960 | ISBN 9781572848498 (ebook)
Subjects: LCSH: Athletes--Nutrition. | Cooking (Natural foods) | Vegan
    cooking. | LCGFT: Cookbooks.
Classification: LCC TX361.A8 A74 2021  (print) | LCC TX361.A8
(ebook) |
    DDC 641.5/6362--dc23
LC record available at https://lccn.loc.gov/2020040118
LC ebook record available at https://lccn.loc.gov/2020040119

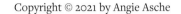

10  9  8  7  6  5  4  3  2          21  22  23  24  25

Art direction and cover design by Morgan Krehbiel
Cover photo by Katie Hass
Interior photography by Katie Hass and Casey Haley

Agate books are available in bulk at discount prices.
For more information, visit agatepublishing.com.

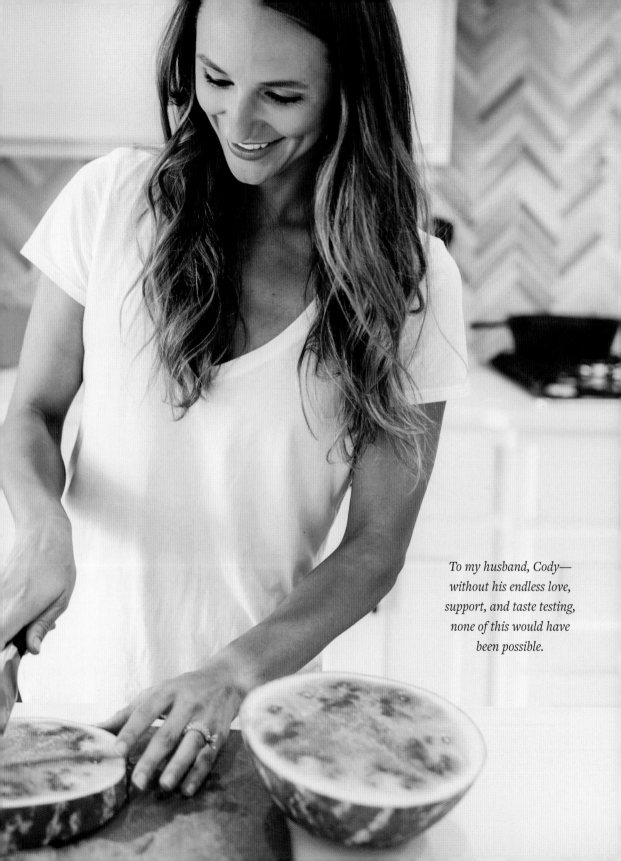

*To my husband, Cody—
without his endless love,
support, and taste testing,
none of this would have
been possible.*

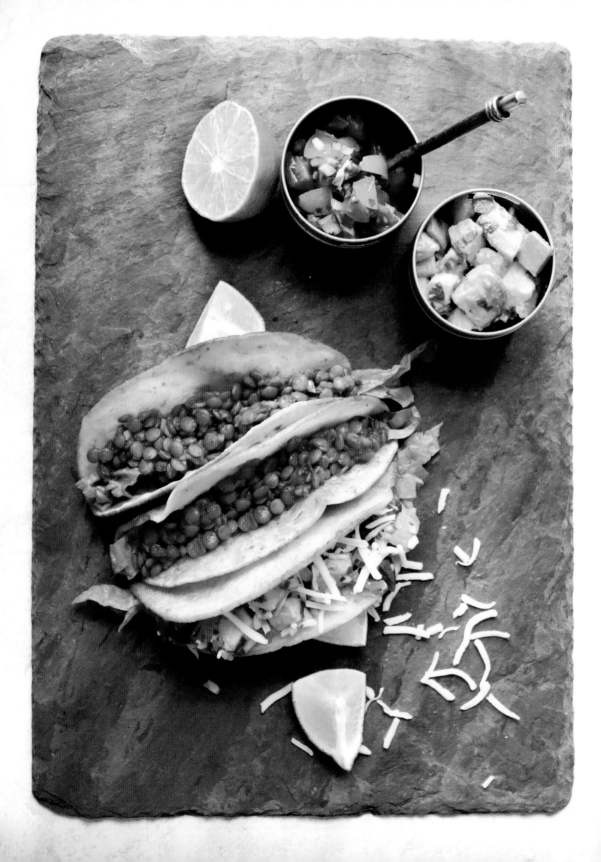

# CONTENTS

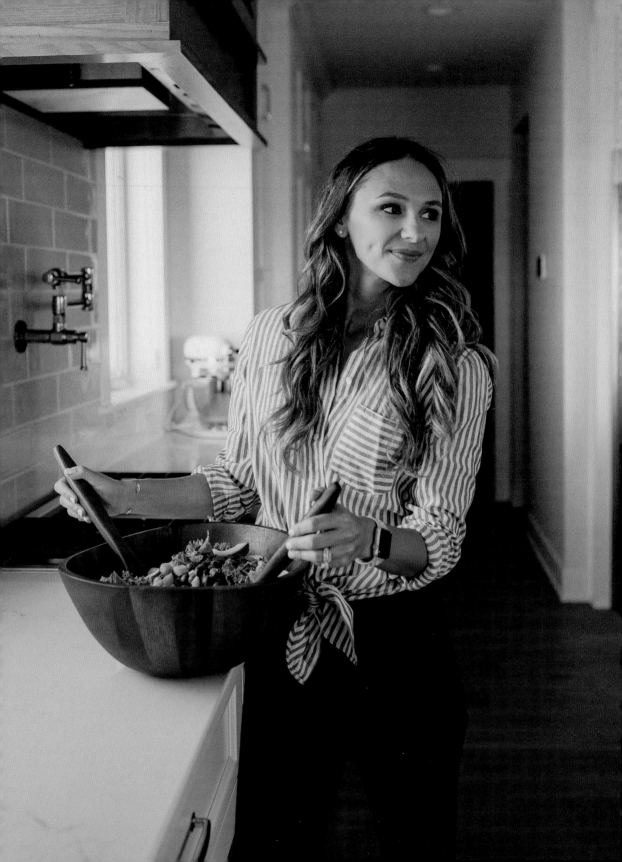

# INTRODUCTION
## WHY ATHLETES NEED THIS BOOK

**F**ROM MY PROFESSIONAL EXPERIENCE consulting athletes across the country to my personal experience being married to one, I have seen firsthand the challenges that high-performance athletes face. Between training and competition—especially if that includes travel—cooking time and kitchen space are often limited. The majority of the athletes I meet with for the first time lack the knowledge and understanding of just how crucial proper nutrition is for optimal performance. They may also lack confidence in the kitchen or the knowledge of basic cooking skills. However, these athletes tend to be eager to learn about nutrition and how to cook nourishing recipes. And if you are reading this, I know you are, too.

Growing up as a competitive dancer and swimmer, I was always intrigued by the impact certain foods had on my performance. When I was still in high school, I was fortunate enough to shadow dietitians to learn more about sports nutrition. My passion for science grew, and I started to learn how and why foods can be either beneficial or detrimental to performance and overall health. Throughout college, I worked as a certified personal trainer and quickly realized that an exercise program alone is not enough to optimize performance.

So I decided to take an uncommon path. I graduated college with bachelor's degrees in both exercise science and dietetics, completed a master's degree in nutrition and physical performance, and became both a registered dietitian and a certified exercise physiologist. Combining the studies of exercise science and dietetics gave me a powerhouse of specialized knowledge that I could apply to every classification of athlete. I wanted to offer my clients something more than other nutritionists or health coaches could. As a board-certified sports dietitian, I provide evidence-based nutrition guidance and strategies to enhance lifelong health, fitness, and sports performance.

Unfortunately, not everyone has access to consult one-on-one with a professional sports dietitian. Moreover, the internet is full of conflicting information about what and how to eat to improve performance, and it can be challenging for anyone to sift through it all to find effective fueling strategies. It became my dream to create a resource that demystifies performance nutrition and cooking for athletes who train at a high level—whether amateurs, professionals, retired, or just starting out—and I'm overjoyed to finally be able to share this with the world.

The decision to sit down and write this book came directly from my athletes. Countless times, athletes have asked me for book recommendations on two main topics: (1) nutrition for improving athletic performance and recovery and (2) recipes and cookbooks geared toward athletes.

Sure, I could suggest several academic books on sports nutrition, but these were often overwhelming to athletes just wanting a good understanding of the basics, not the physiological breakdown of the adenosine triphosphate–phosphocreatine (ATP-PC) system. As for cookbooks, there were plenty I could recommend, but most on the market were geared specifically toward endurance athletes, and that type of information does not align with the needs of *all* performance athletes, whose nutrition goals are varied and may change throughout a season or career. Consider the minor league baseball player living in an extended-stay hotel room, the college football player trying to gain 15 pounds over an off-season, or the competitive figure skater needing quick and simple recipes after 8-plus hours at the rink.

I wanted to fill this void by combining my sports nutrition knowledge, experience working with athletes, and nutritious recipes into an all-in-one book—a comprehensive resource to help all active people better understand what and when to eat to help maximize performance on and off the field (or court or rink). Whether you are an athlete at the recreational or elite level, the foods you choose to eat have a direct impact on your overall health, performance, and recovery. This book shows you what to eat, why you should eat it, and how to cook it.

Educating athletes about what foods are beneficial to their health and performance is obviously crucial. But what is often neglected in sports nutrition education is the next step: teaching them how to cook and prepare these foods with limited time and resources. You don't need years of experience to cook delicious, nourishing meals, and this book is here to walk you through the basics. What I've found is that athletes are eager to cook for themselves; they simply lack the know-how, the time, or both. These meals are meant for the busiest individuals, with symbols directing you toward recipes that take 30 minutes or less or recipes you can make even if you don't have access to a fully equipped kitchen.

My nutrition philosophy emphasizes an anti-inflammatory diet. By placing a priority on whole-food nutrition, I aim to promote recovery, decrease inflammation, and improve overall health. I've included sample meal plans for weight management, weight gain, and vegan/vegetarian athletes, along with nutritional information for each recipe. *Fuel Your Body* provides a roadmap for selecting meals that fit your unique situation and dietary needs. Throughout this book, symbols are included to direct you toward recipes that are dairy-free, gluten-free, nut-free, vegan, and/or vegetarian.

Understanding performance nutrition can be overwhelming, especially if you lack the skills or confidence to prepare meals on your own. *Fuel Your Body* solves this problem. At its core, this book is about helping you feel confident preparing nourishing meals and providing you with plenty of healthy recipes for even the busiest athletes. Now let's get started!

> Educating athletes about what foods are beneficial to their health and performance is obviously crucial. But what is often neglected in sports nutrition education is the next step: **teaching them how to cook and prepare these foods with limited time and resources.**

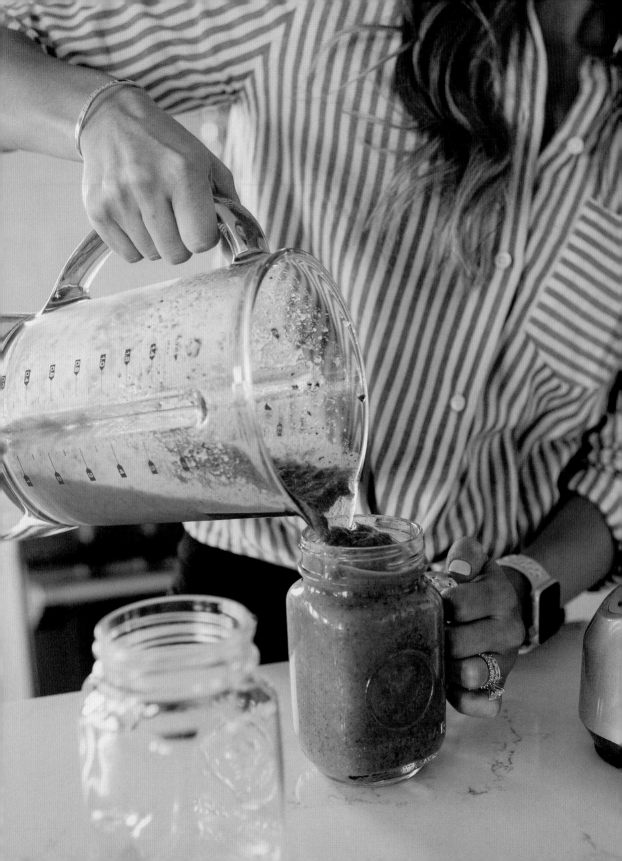

# PART ONE

## PERFORMANCE NUTRITION BASICS

## CHAPTER ONE

# PERFORMANCE NUTRITION

P erformance nutrition, also referred to as sports nutrition, is the study and field of nutrition with the goal of improving athletic performance. The focus of performance nutrition is the right types of foods, in the right amounts, and at the right times in order to optimize training ability and recovery. Put simply, nutrition is essential for athletes as it provides the source of energy necessary to perform. In other words, **food** is **fuel**.

Anyone with a physically active lifestyle, regardless of whether they are a competitive athlete or an avid gym-goer, can benefit from implementing aspects of performance nutrition. I use the term *athlete* often in this book. Keep in mind that when I use this term, I am referring to anyone who competes in a sport *or* who is habitually physically active. Performance nutrition is not one-size-fits-all, and an individual's lifestyle, sport or activity, personal goals, and/or medical condition can all lead to variations in nutrient needs. Reading through this book in its entirety will help you figure out what's right for you.

This chapter discusses the three macronutrients: carbohydrates, protein, and fat. It then covers what's called *nutrient timing*, the ideal timing of your meals to best optimize performance and recovery. Finally, it provides a breakdown of supplements, followed by steps to calculate your energy needs, as well as the importance of implementing "nourishment over numbers."

# THE MACRONUTRIENTS

Macronutrients are the three types of nutrients that your body requires in large amounts: carbohydrates, protein, and fat. Macronutrients provide your body with energy (calories), and all three play crucial roles in making sure your body is functioning at its best. While most foods contain multiple macronutrients, they are typically categorized by the macronutrient that they contain the most of. For example, rice and potatoes are often categorized as carbohydrates, even though they do contain small amounts of protein. And beef and salmon are often categorized as proteins, but they do both contain fat as well. Let's discuss each macronutrient individually to learn why all three are important for your overall health and performance.

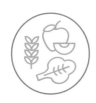

### CARBOHYDRATES

Carbohydrates are the body's most efficient source of energy. When carbs are consumed, the body converts them to glucose, which then provides an immediate energy source for all forms of exercise. Glycogen, the body's stored form of carbohydrates, is used during high-intensity exercise to provide both power and speed. Intense exercise depletes glycogen stores, which are then restored by consuming more carbohydrates. When you do not consume adequate carbs, you run the risk of poor concentration and focus, a decrease in performance, and a breakdown of lean muscle mass as a fuel source. There are numerous myths surrounding carbohydrates and performance, which I address in my nutrition myths section (see page 34).

How many carbohydrates do you need? The amount of carbohydrates an athlete should consume varies significantly depending on the activity, level of intensity, and duration, ranging from 3 to 12 grams per kilogram of body weight per day. This is a very wide range, because when it comes to energy expenditure, there are many differences even within the same sport. The athlete's position, weight, body composition goals, and even where they're at in their training cycle all affect carbohydrate needs. For example, a starting pitcher burns significantly more calories than an outfielder, but also starts only once every five days. In football, a cornerback and a defensive tackle both play defense, but they likely have very different body sizes and composition, making carbohydrate requirements extremely variable depending on the individual.

A very generalized guideline is that athletes performing at moderate to high intensities, or training 1 to 3 hours per day, should aim for at least 5 to 8 grams of carbs per kilogram of body weight per day. For athletes training at very high intensities and for very long durations (for example, long-distance runners), carbohydrate recommendations go up to 8 to 12 grams per kilogram of body weight per day. Carb-loading is a common practice in endurance athletes in the days leading up to a race. By increasing carbohydrate intake to 8 to 12 grams per kilogram of body weight in the final 72 hours leading up to a prolonged endurance competition, athletes can increase muscle glycogen stores, especially when training volume is tapered back. Increased muscle glycogen stores may help athletes exercise harder for longer, as it helps delay the onset of muscle fatigue.

Carbohydrates are the body's preferred source of energy, so it is very important for athletes to adjust their carb intake before, during, and after hard training sessions to ensure adequate replenishment. Some general guidelines are to consume 1 to 2 grams of carbs per kilogram of body weight 1 to 2 hours before exercise. For endurance exercise that will last longer than 60 to 90 minutes (such as running), a general guideline is to consume 30 to 60 grams of carbohydrates per hour during exercise. For optimal recovery post-workout, a general guideline is to aim for up to 1.5 grams of carbs per kilogram of body weight right after you finish exercising, and then continue to replenish with carbohydrates throughout the day. Although protein also plays a very important role in repairing muscle, without adequate carbohydrates, the recovery process is not as efficient.

Carbohydrates are found in a wide variety of foods. You might have heard that simple carbs are "bad" and complex carbs are "good," but for athletes, the type of carbs you should eat depends on what you're doing. Simple carbohydrates are sugars (such as fructose and glucose) that are easy for your body to break down. They are absorbed quickly and can provide you with a jolt of energy. That's why they can come in handy mid-competition, when your glycogen stores are running low and you need an immediate source of glucose.

Honey Stinger Waffles, GU energy gels, gummies, jelly beans, and sports drinks like Gatorade are just a few of the many products athletes often use mid-competition for an energy boost. However, simple carbohydrates should account for only a small amount of your carb intake, and they should be utilized only when necessary.

Instead, most of your carbs should come from complex carbohydrates, which have a more complicated molecular structure that takes the body longer to break down. Often, though not always, complex carbs are found in whole foods with fiber, vitamins, minerals, and sometimes protein and/or fat. Whole-food sources of complex carbs, such as orange slices, bananas, and even cooked potatoes, are all options athletes can use in place of traditional products mid-competition.

In general, the best sources of carbohydrates are whole, unprocessed foods, such as vegetables, fruits, oats, rice, whole-grain pasta, whole-grain bread, beans, lentils, and potatoes. It's best to stay away from processed foods that provide energy (calories) but not much nutritional value (vitamins, minerals, fiber, protein, fat). Some examples include refined white flour, cane sugar, fruit juice, and soda.

What about keto or low-carb diets for athletes? It's true that training with limited carbohydrate availability can lead to an increase in fat utilization during training, meaning that your body may shift in favor of using more fat as fuel than carbohydrates. However, there's insufficient evidence supporting a performance benefit, and research continues to show that training with limited carbohydrate availability impairs intensity and duration. When your body is training at moderate intensities—if, say, you are an ultra runner sustaining the same intensity through a prolonged endurance event—your body is more capable of oxidizing fat for fuel. But at higher intensities or for high-intensity intermittent sports, such as hockey, basketball, and soccer, carbohydrates are the preferred energy source, and performance is impaired when intake is low.

### PROTEIN

Protein helps build and repair the body's tissues. It is vital for the health of your skin, hair, bones, muscles, cartilage, and even for the production of red blood cells. Protein is composed of 20 amino acids. Only half of these amino acids can be produced by the body; the other half, known as essential amino acids, must be consumed from the foods we eat. Just as carbohydrate needs vary depending on certain factors, so do protein needs. Athletes who undergo intense training (that is, exercising at maximum or very hard effort) daily need more than twice as much protein as recommended by the US National Institutes of Health for the general population. So while the current recommended dietary allowance (RDA) is just 0.8 grams per kilogram of body weight per day, this should be doubled for athletes, to closer to 1.6 to 2.0 grams per kilogram of body weight per day.

For athletes trying to decrease body fat while preventing loss of lean muscle mass, I recommend consuming between 2.0 and 2.4 grams of protein per kilogram of body weight per day. For vegans and vegetarians, I recommend at least 1.6 grams per kilogram of body weight per day due to plant protein's lower bioavailability (that is, the body's ability to absorb and utilize). Contrary to popular belief, protein can be found in numerous plant foods, such as soy products, beans, lentils, nuts, and seeds. Several recipes in this cookbook are based on these plant protein sources. I've also designed a meal plan (see page 52) for vegan and vegetarian athletes, and for those of you wanting to try eating a more plant-based diet. A plant-based diet is linked to a lower risk of heart disease, diabetes, and certain cancers. You've probably heard a recommendation to include a variety of fruits and vegetables in your diet; the same goes for plant-based proteins. Consuming a variety of protein-rich plant foods (such as lentils, black beans, peas, chickpeas, quinoa, tempeh, and tofu) throughout the day will help ensure that you obtain the protein and essential amino acids your body needs.

Whenever I'm discussing protein with clients, two questions almost always come up: "What are BCAAs?" and "What about collagen protein?" Branched-chain amino acids, or BCAAs, are three essential amino acids: leucine, isoleucine, and valine. What makes them unique is that they are the only amino acids that can be utilized by the muscles as fuel. Leucine has been shown to be especially beneficial in stimulating muscle protein synthesis, or the repairing and building of muscle. If you eat eggs, dairy, fish, poultry, or meat, or if you use a whey- or plant-based protein powder (see Supplements, page 19), you're likely consuming adequate BCAAs, so additional supplementation isn't necessary. And contrary to popular belief, BCAA supplements are no more effective than the amino acids found naturally in food sources.

Collagen is a crucial component of connective tissue, cartilage, bone, and skin. As the popularity of collagen supplements continues to grow, you may wonder whether this is a protein source you should be adding to your diet. Collagen supplements are sourced from animal bones, skin, and connective tissues. When you consume them, your body breaks them down into amino acids, then synthesizes its own collagen from there. In fact, your body actually produces collagen naturally on a daily basis by using vitamin C and amino acids (glycine and proline) to create procollagen molecules.

While the research is slim on collagen supplementation for athletes specifically, it is promising in terms of skin and joint health. Collagen supplementation in combination with vitamin C has been shown to help strengthen ligaments and tendons. Collagen also seems to be beneficial for reducing symptoms associated with osteoarthritis and for aiding in recovery post–ACL injury.

If you'd like to supplement with collagen, consider it an addition to otherwise high-quality protein sources rather than a replacement. While potentially beneficial for joint health, collagen is actually not considered a complete protein source as it lacks an essential amino acid. You can also consume collagen from whole-food sources, such as bone broth and eggs. In addition to these whole-food sources, minimizing your intake of highly processed foods, staying hydrated, and consuming a diet rich in antioxidants, omega-3 fatty acids, and vitamins A and C will help your body produce collagen naturally.

### FAT

Fat provides energy, helps protect cell membranes throughout the body, and plays a crucial role in regulating hormones. Fat also allows the body to absorb fat-soluble vitamins (A, D, E, and K), and certain fats may help fight disease and inflammation. For years, dietary fat was assumed to be evil. Fat was assumed to "make you fat" and was believed to be the culprit of high cholesterol and heart disease. Though this idea was long ago debunked, fat-free and nonfat "diet" products still fill the supermarket shelves, egg white omelets are still found under the "healthy choices" section of restaurant menus, and reduced-fat peanut butter is still very much a thing. Truth is, fat is essential. Diets where fat makes up less than 15 percent of total caloric intake can result in deficiencies of essential fatty acids and/or fat-soluble vitamins and can contribute to menstrual dysfunction in female athletes.

You should aim to consume around 1 gram of fat per kilogram of body weight per day. Unsaturated fats (monounsaturated and polyunsaturated) should make up the majority of your fat intake. Examples include extra-virgin olive oil, nuts and nut butters, seeds, avocados, avocado oil, and fatty fish. Trans fats, which are found in partially hydrogenated oils, margarine, and highly processed foods, should be excluded from your diet. Trans fats are known to increase low-density lipoprotein (LDL) cholesterol, which raises the risk for heart disease. Conversely, unsaturated fats help increase high-density lipoprotein (HDL) cholesterol, which can decrease the risk for heart disease.

Omega-3 fatty acids are also an important part of your diet. Omega-3s play crucial roles in enhancing brain function, promoting growth and development, and reducing inflammation. They are essential fatty acids, meaning they can't be produced by the body and must be consumed. The three most important omega-3 fatty acids are docosahexaenoic acid (DHA) and eicosapentaenoic acid (EPA), both of which are found in fish and shellfish, and alpha-linolenic acid (ALA), which is found in plants. For athletes who don't eat seafood regularly, consuming plant sources of ALA like flaxseed, chia seeds, and walnuts is a great way to obtain more omega-3s.

In a research collaboration by the Collegiate and Professional Sports Dietitians Association (CPSDA), researchers found that most college athletes were consuming only 35 percent of the recommended 2 grams of omega-3s each day. As with most nutrients, it's better to get them from whole foods than supplements, since whole foods provide additional nutrients. If you enjoy fish, try consuming 8 ounces of fatty fish per week, and aim for a variety—salmon, mackerel, herring, and albacore tuna. The benefits of consuming these nutritious foods outweighs taking an omega-3 supplement, as just one serving of salmon also provides you with vitamin D, protein, and several B vitamins. Likewise, for plant sources, in one serving of flaxseed oil you also consume fiber, protein, and magnesium.

# PRE-WORKOUT NUTRITION

It's important to understand the types of foods you should be consuming in the hours leading up to your workout because what you choose to eat can either help or hinder your performance. It's also important that you learn through your own trial and error which foods and fluids work best for you personally; no single meal or snack is going to work for everyone.

> It's important to learn which foods and fluids work best for you personally; no single meal or snack is going to work for everyone.

If you're able to consume a meal several hours before a hard training session or competition, this can consist of all three macronutrients—carbohydrates, protein, and fat—with an emphasis on carbohydrates and protein. For larger meals, allow 3 to 5 hours to digest; for smaller meals, allow 2 to 3 hours; and for small snacks or liquids such as smoothies (see page 69), allow up to 1 hour. As you get closer to game time or your training session (see the illustration on page 15), the amount of recommended protein and fat starts to taper off. Right before a workout, you should eat primarily carbohydrates, small to moderate amounts of protein, and limited fat.

Your pre-workout or pregame meal could be grilled or baked chicken or fish with wild rice or whole-grain pasta with a mixed green salad. If the pregame meal comes at breakfast time, this could be a bowl of muesli (see page 86) with a banana or a vegetable omelet with whole-grain toast and fresh fruit. Your pre-workout meal should contain at least 20 grams of protein and 2 grams of leucine.

Fiber intake may also need to be limited, especially in the hour leading up to your event. Too much fat or fiber immediately before a workout can lead to gastrointestinal upset (bloating, gas, and cramping). This will vary depending on the individual and how much fiber they consume overall in their diet. For example, an athlete who normally consumes a high-fiber diet might not have any problem including fiber in their pre-workout meal. However, an athlete who has irritable bowel syndrome (IBS) or who typically consumes a lower-fiber diet may experience gastrointestinal issues.

Consuming adequate carbohydrates pre-workout can help maintain normal blood sugar levels, prevent hunger mid-workout, and provide enough energy to fuel your muscles. Specific amounts of carbohydrates will vary depending on the athlete, but a general guideline is to consume 1 gram of carbs per kilogram of body weight 1 hour before training. Convenient options include a slice of bread topped with peanut butter, sliced bananas, and honey; half of a peanut butter and banana sandwich; Greek yogurt with granola and berries; or a granola bar.

To stay on top of your hydration, drink at least 16 to 24 ounces of fluid 2 hours before your workout, followed by an additional 8 ounces of fluid in the 30 minutes leading up to your workout.

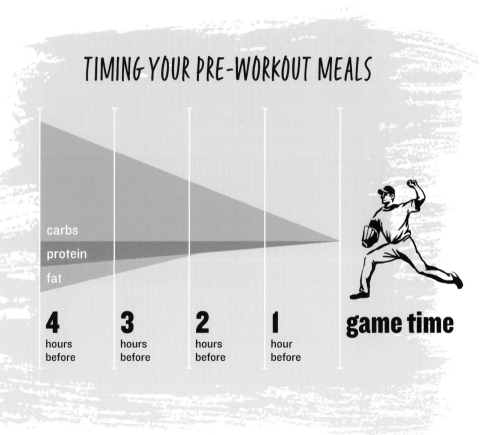

TIMING YOUR PRE-WORKOUT MEALS

carbs
protein
fat

**4** hours before   **3** hours before   **2** hours before   **1** hour before   **game time**

# HYDRATING YOUR WORKOUT

Did you know that hockey players can lose as much as 1.8 liters of fluid, and goalies over 3 liters, during a single practice? A 2 percent loss in body weight (for example, a 4-pound loss in a 200-pound athlete) is defined as dehydration; a 3 percent loss (a 6-pound loss in a 200-pound athlete) can significantly impair performance.

Common sweat rates range from 1 to 4 pounds per hour and vary depending on exercise intensity, duration, heat, humidity, and altitude. One way to stay on top of your hydration needs and estimated sweat rate is by weighing yourself before and immediately after your training session, while also keeping track of how many ounces of fluid you consumed. For each pound you lost in sweat, aim to consume 16 to 24 ounces of fluid after your workout. Sweat contains electrolytes, primarily sodium and lesser amounts of potassium. Try incorporating sodium- and potassium-rich foods in the meals and snacks leading up to your training session or competition, and continue to replace electrolytes lost during your workout through electrolyte products or sports drinks, such as my Homemade Sports Drinks (see page 186).

> Common sweat rates range from 1 to 4 pounds per hour and vary depending on exercise intensity, duration, heat, humidity, and altitude.

Hydration isn't the only thing to monitor during your workout; you must keep your energy level up, too. Your glycogen stores can become depleted after about 90 minutes of intense exercise. This can lead to early fatigue, reduced training intensity, decreased performance. and increased risk of injury. For workouts lasting longer than 90 minutes, consume 30 to 60 grams of carbohydrates per hour. Whether these carbohydrates come in the form of a sports drink, a gel, a banana, or even a granola bar, your snack should be individualized based on your personal preference and what your stomach can tolerate. For ultra-endurance exercise lasting 3 hours or longer, higher intakes of carbohydrates are necessary, up to 90 grams per hour.

# POST-WORKOUT NUTRITION

Adequate nutrition after a hard training session or competition is just as important as what you eat before. Your goals should be to refuel, repair your muscles, and replenish your body for your next training session. To recover quickly, aim to consume adequate carbohydrates, protein, and fluid within the first hour after your workout.

Glycogen is restored by consuming carbohydrates. After intense exercise, aim for 1.5 grams per kilogram of body weight, then an additional 1.5 grams per kilogram of body weight 2 hours later. To help repair muscle tissue and reduce muscle breakdown, you should also consume at least 15 to 25 grams of protein within the first hour.

Some athletes experience a loss of appetite after intense training sessions. This is because when we exercise, we experience a decrease in ghrelin, the hormone that makes us feel hungry, and an increase in peptide YY, the hormone that is responsible for suppressing our appetite and making us feel satiated. This is especially common immediately after cardiovascular exercise, such as running. If you're someone who experiences a poor appetite post-workout, it may be challenging to consume adequate carbohydrates and protein for your body to recover. Smoothies, such as the Chocolate-Banana Smoothie (see page 78), are a good solution, as they provide carbohydrates, protein, and fluids all in one. Protein powders are handy for athletes who don't have much of an appetite after working out because they can easily be blended into a smoothie or used to make Post-Workout Recovery Bites (see page 184).

If you plan to eat a balanced meal within about an hour of finishing your training session, this could be your recovery meal. But if it will be several hours and you're needing a quick recovery snack beforehand, make sure to plan ahead and pack these snacks with you. A few examples include Endurance Trail Mix (see page 190) and 3-Ingredient Energy Bars (see page 187). The following illustration shows additional food options that contain carbohydrates, protein, fluids, or a combination.

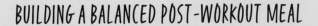

# BUILDING A BALANCED POST-WORKOUT MEAL

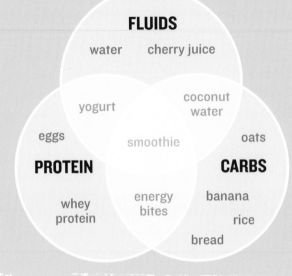

**FLUIDS**

water    cherry juice

yogurt    coconut water

eggs    smoothie    oats

**PROTEIN**    **CARBS**

whey protein    energy bites    banana

rice

bread

### HOW CAN DRINKING ALCOHOL AFTER A WORKOUT AFFECT PERFORMANCE?

After exercise, it's important to replenish glycogen stores and stimulate muscle protein synthesis. That's why consuming carbohydrates and protein is recommended. However, when you consume alcohol after a workout, that delays the recovery process by decreasing muscle protein synthesis and interfering with glycogen replenishment. This can make it very difficult to boost performance and muscle growth over time. Alcohol also impairs hydration status, which can affect the quality and duration of your next workout. If you're recovering from an injury, research shows that consuming alcohol could prolong recovery time. Studies have indicated that two to three alcoholic drinks per day impairs testosterone levels by decreasing secretion, which can impair protein synthesis and negatively affect the results from resistance training over time. Your post-workout focus should be on consuming a carbohydrate- and protein-rich meal, and allowing enough time to digest and recover, before drinking a beer or cocktail.

# SUPPLEMENTS

The US Food and Drug Administration (FDA) does not regulate supplements; instead, they go through what's called post-market approval. This means that anyone can legally make and sell supplements without a single clinical trial, without having to prove that what's on the label is actually in the product, and without having to do any background checks as far as sanitation or cross-contamination at the manufacturing facility. As long as a supplement company isn't stating that its produce will cure a disease, it can pretty much make any claim it wants. This is why it's so important for anyone using supplements, both athletes and nonathletes, to use products that are verified through a quality assurance company such as United States Pharmacopeia (USP) or National Sanitation Foundation (NSF). For athletes specifically, I recommend using only those products that carry the third-party certification "NSF Certified for Sport" or "Informed Sport." These certifications assure that what's listed on the package is what's actually in the product.

The most common supplements I recommend to athletes are creatine, omega-3s, vitamin D, and protein powder. Let's break them down.

**Creatine.** Creatine is a molecule synthesized in the body by amino acids such as glycine and methionine. While creatine can be produced by the body, it is also found naturally in food sources, mainly meat and seafood. About 95 percent of creatine is stored in the body's muscles as phosphocreatine. Think of phosphocreatine as the energy needed for very short, high-intensity exercises like sprints. When you supplement with creatine, you are increasing the stores of phosphocreatine within your muscles anywhere from 10 to 40 percent, allowing your body to be able to work at a higher intensity for a longer period of time. Creatine can improve sprint performance, maximize strength and power, and have positive effects on lean body mass. Creatine is ideal for athletes who train with explosiveness, power, and strength and who consistently train at high intensities and utilize weight training. In addition, vegan and vegetarian athletes may greatly benefit from creatine supplementation, as these athletes in particular tend to have low phosphocreatine stores. Creatine supplements have been heavily researched and are considered safe; the recommended dose is 3 to 5 grams per day in the form of creatine monohydrate.

**Omega-3s.** As discussed earlier (see page 13), omega-3 fatty acids have numerous health benefits. If you have a hard time consuming enough omega-3s in your diet, supplementation may be necessary. Nordic Naturals and Klean Athlete are two companies that offer an NSF Certified for Sport omega-3 fish oil supplement.

**Protein powder.** While definitely not a necessity, protein powder is a convenient and quickly digested source of protein, which can be especially handy for athletes who are traveling. Whey protein powder is sourced from milk, while vegan protein powders contain a blend of different plant proteins, most often pea and brown rice. For athletes who have a hard time consuming solid food after working out, protein powders are a great option. Adding one scoop to a smoothie will also provide the optimal 20 grams of protein and 2 grams of leucine recommended post-workout.

**Vitamin D.** This vitamin works to maximize the absorption of calcium, aids in bone mineralization, and helps protect against fractures. Vitamin D is less abundant in food sources beyond fortified milk, egg yolks, salmon, and cod liver oil. Because sun exposure is a main source of vitamin D, athletes who train primarily indoors or live in areas of the country with little sun exposure could be at higher risk of developing a vitamin D deficiency. Micronutrient deficiencies and specific recommendations as far as dosages should be determined by your healthcare provider.

As far as all supplements are concerned, it's preferable to obtain the necessary nutrients from whole-food sources, but this is simply not realistic for some athletes. For example, athletes with a history of stress fractures, bone or joint injuries, or little exposure to sunlight can be at increased risk of low vitamin D levels, and diet alone usually does not prove effective. If an athlete has multiple food allergies, this could also make it challenging to meet nutrient needs through food alone. And for athletes who eat a vegan or vegetarian diet, the main nutrients of concern are vitamin B12, iron, zinc, calcium, omega-3s, and protein.

Supplementation should be individualized to the athlete based on their specific needs; a sports dietitian can help determine the most appropriate options for you.

## WHAT ABOUT PROBIOTICS?

Probiotics are living microorganisms (bacteria and yeasts) that provide health benefits such as improved digestion and immune function. Often referred to as "good" gut bacteria, probiotics are found in fermented foods such as yogurt, kimchi, miso, kefir, tempeh, and sauerkraut. Probiotics work best when taken in tandem with prebiotics, which are essentially indigestible carbohydrates, also known as fiber, that feed the healthy bacteria in the gut. Fruit, vegetables, beans, and whole grains are rich sources of fiber. Including food sources that contain both probiotics and prebiotics will lead to the most overall benefit to your gut health.

Probiotics may be especially beneficial for athletes with IBS or ulcerative colitis, or who are just coming off a course of antibiotics. More recent research also suggests that probiotics may be beneficial in reducing the incidence of upper respiratory infections (such as the common cold) in athletes. However, numerous questions remain unanswered regarding which strains are best and how the effectiveness of supplements compares to whole fermented food sources. I recommend incorporating more probiotic-rich food sources into your diet before adding a probiotic supplement.

# ESTIMATING YOUR ENERGY NEEDS

Nearly every athlete I work with comes to me with a body composition goal in mind. Typically, these athletes want to lose fat, gain lean muscle mass, or make weight for a specific event. They often tell me that they estimated their energy needs using an online calorie calculator. Unfortunately, it doesn't seem that many of these calculators were designed with the needs of athletes in mind.

Athletes tend to have a higher percentage of lean muscle mass than non-athletes, which results in a higher basal metabolic rate (BMR) than estimated by online calculators, since muscle burns more at rest than fat. These calculators also don't take into account an athlete's training cycle, often referred to as periodization. Depending on where you're at in your training cycle—for instance, if you're in the middle of your season versus the off-season—your energy needs will vary. Just as your training intensity and volume will change throughout your competition cycle, your nutrition should change as well. This can be referred to as "nutrition periodization."

When an athlete comes to me struggling to gain weight, I can usually assume that they aren't consuming enough calories. But what often shocks athletes is when they come to me for weight loss and I tell them that they, too, aren't consuming enough calories. Athletes who do not consume enough energy (that is, calories) to meet their body's needs often end up with unwanted loss of muscle mass, hormonal imbalances, menstrual dysfunction, suboptimal bone density, and an increased risk of fatigue, illness, and injury. All the risks resulting from low energy availability have a negative impact not only on performance but on overall health.

To know if you're eating enough, you'll need to take a close look at the nutritional content of the foods you consume. For at least five days, keep a food journal of everything you eat and drink, then meet with a sports dietitian to review. It's crucial to correctly analyze your current nutrition and see where you may be falling short in terms of macronutrients (carbohydrates, fat, protein) and micronutrients (vitamins, minerals).

To do so, first you'll need to calculate your resting metabolic rate (RMR). Your RMR is approximately how many calories your body burns at rest. This will give you an estimate of how many calories your body needs to function optimally on your nontraining or rest days. To get an accurate measurement of an athlete's RMR, I have the individual breathe directly into a tube on a machine called an indirect calorimeter. The machine is then able to collect and measure the oxygen their body consumes to accurately measure their RMR. But you can get a rough estimate of your RMR at home by using the Cunningham equation, shown below. It's often used for athletes because it focuses on lean body mass (LBM) as opposed to total body weight.

**CUNNINGHAM EQUATION**
500 + (22 × LBM) = estimated RMR

**TO CALCULATE LBM:**
body fat (%) × total body weight (kg) = fat mass (kg)
total body weight (kg) – fat mass (kg) = LBM

Now that you have your estimated RMR, you need to multiply it by the activity factor that most resembles your current training regimen:

| Low: | **1.2** | *little to no training* |
|---|---|---|
| Light: | **1.375** | *light exercise or sport 1 to 3 days per week* |
| Moderate: | **1.55** | *moderate exercise or sport 6 to 7 days per week* |
| High: | **1.725** | *hard training or exercise daily* |
| Very High: | **1.9** | *extremely active, hard training 2 or more times per day* |

This will yield the number of calories you should be taking in each day during this period. There is another step, however: adding or subtracting calories in small amounts to accommodate your goal of either weight gain or weight loss. If your goal is to gain weight, I typically recommend adding another 500 calories to allow for consistent weight gain. For weight loss, I usually recommend that athletes start by subtracting only 250 calories to allow for consistent weight loss without negatively impacting performance or risking loss of lean body mass. Increasing protein intake is also important when weight loss is your goal; I recommend at least 2 grams per kilogram of body weight per day.

The recipes in this cookbook are meant to be used by all athletes, regardless of your body composition goals. Nutritional information for each recipe is found at the back of the book (see page 216). You can also try my weight gain and weight management sample meal plans if you need a little more structure (see page 43). Please note that these are samples, so they're not individualized to your specific needs.

If you've been trying to make changes to your weight but have been unsuccessful, keep in mind that other factors besides exercise can play a role in increasing or decreasing your energy needs. Factors that increase energy needs include exposure to excessive cold or heat, high altitudes, stress, physical injuries, increase in lean body mass, certain drugs and medications, and possibly the luteal phase of the menstrual cycle. Factors that decrease energy needs include aging, decrease in lean body mass, and possibly the follicular phase of the menstrual cycle.

# A CLOSER LOOK AT CALCULATING DAILY CALORIES

Let's calculate the estimated daily calorie intake for a sample athlete we'll call Mark. Mark is a 6'3", 160-pound (**72 kg**), 18-year-old baseball player. His body fat is **10 percent**, and his activity factor is described as **high**, considering he trains hard every day. He wants to **gain 20 pounds**.

▷ First, to calculate Mark's fat mass, we multiply his body fat by his total body weight (in kilograms): **0.10 × 72 = 7.2 kg**

▷ Next, we calculate his LBM, by subtracting his fat mass from his total body weight: **72 − 7.2 = 64.8 kg**

▷ Now we can calculate his RMR using the Cunningham equation: **500 + (22 x 64.8) = 1,925 calories/day**

▷ Finally, we multiply his RMR by his high activity factor, which is 1.725: **1,925 × 1.725 = 3,320 calories/day**

Thus, Mark needs to take in 3,320 calories per day to maintain his current weight at his current activity level. But Mark's goal is to gain 20 pounds, so I recommend that he add another 500 calories per day to allow for consistent weight gain: **3,320 + 500 = 3,820 calories/day**

This is the number of calories Mark should aim for in order to gain weight while training at a high level.

## NOURISHMENT OVER NUMBERS

Food is so much more than grams of carbs, fat, and protein. When we focus on nourishment over numbers, we make better choices. How is this food nourishing me? What kind of nutrients does it contain—vitamins, minerals, omega-3s, fiber? But food can be nourishing in other ways, too. A food item that is not particularly rich in nutrients might nourish you mentally or socially. Ask yourself: Am I truly enjoying this food? Food is nourishment for your mental and emotional health. Think of all the memories you have with family or friends that involve food. Are there certain dishes that bring you back to a pleasant childhood memory or a new cultural experience? Making it a point to incorporate foods that bring you joy is just as important for your overall health.

There's a reason the nutritional information for my recipes is collected at the back of this book and not front and center on every recipe. Athletes often get so caught up in tracking macros or counting calories that they lose sight of what's really important: nourishment. They become so obsessed with numbers that they overthink their food choices and ignore their body's nutritional needs—both physically and mentally. They may choose a food solely based on it being low-carb or low-calorie, without acknowledging how nutrient-dense that food really is. A great example of a nutrient-dense food is an avocado. While an avocado contains over 300 calories, it also boasts over 900 mg potassium, 13 g fiber, 20 g monounsaturated fats, 4 g protein, 30 percent of the RDA of vitamin C, and 15 percent of the RDA of magnesium. Compare this to a highly processed 100-calorie snack bar that may boast that it is low-fat or low-carb—it doesn't come close to any of these nutritional values.

Tracking calories or macros absolutely works for some athletes. It helps you control portion sizes and gives you a numerical way to monitor your food intake. It's helped quite a few of my clients get an idea of where they are when they first start working with me, and what areas they need to increase or decrease to reach their goals. But is counting calories or macros necessary to improve your performance? Absolutely not. Food is obviously important, but when thinking about it begins to take over every important thing in our lives, it can truly suck all the joy out of eating and do more harm than good. A preoccupation with food can have negative psychological effects, and the unnecessary guilt that comes from occasionally eating less-healthy foods will impact you more psychologically than it will physically. You can be hitting specific calorie or macronutrient numbers and still be malnourished mentally and emotionally. If this sounds like you, it's important to remind yourself periodically to maintain a balanced attitude about food and avoid focusing solely on the numbers.

## CHAPTER TWO

# FOODS THAT BOOST PERFORMANCE

**N**ow that you know the basics of sports nutrition and the importance of maintaining the proper balance of carbohydrates, protein, and fat when it comes to achieving your performance goals, let's talk more about the nutrients in the foods that you eat. This chapter discusses the importance of an anti-inflammatory diet, as well as several recommended foods to eat regularly for performance and anti-inflammatory benefits. By incorporating these whole-food sources, athletes may strengthen their immune system, prevent injury and illness, minimize fatigue, and recover faster between workouts.

# WHAT IS AN ANTI-INFLAMMATORY DIET?

Chances are pretty high that you've heard the term *anti-inflammatory* being thrown around in the media, without much clarity on what it really means. Put simply, an anti-inflammatory diet is a pattern of eating that prioritizes foods shown to reduce inflammation, such as plant foods rich in antioxidants and omega-3 fatty acids.

Antioxidants fight inflammation by delaying or inhibiting cell damage from free radicals. Free radicals are unstable atoms that may result from essential metabolic processes in the body or be acquired from outside sources such as air pollution and industrial chemicals. They are highly reactive and can attack all kinds of molecules in your body. Fortunately, antioxidants are stable atoms that can neutralize free radicals and reduce their capacity to damage cells. Antioxidants also aid in the growth and repair of injured tissue and can help enhance both short- and long-term recovery from intense exercise. While some antioxidants are produced in the body, others must be consumed through food, the most popular being vitamin C, vitamin E, and beta-carotene.

When your body possesses high amounts of free radicals and low amounts of antioxidants, a condition known as high oxidative stress occurs. Oxidative stress is thought to worsen inflammatory diseases such as rheumatoid arthritis, as well as coronary artery disease and certain neurological disorders.

An anti-inflammatory diet incorporates large amounts of foods rich in antioxidants and omega-3 fatty acids, such as vegetables, fruit, fatty fish (salmon and mackerel), and other monounsaturated fats such as extra-virgin olive oil, avocados, nuts, and seeds. This diet also incorporates whole grains, legumes (beans and lentils), herbs, spices (ginger and turmeric), and herbal teas. Lean cuts of meat and red wine are consumed in moderation (a few times per week), and highly processed foods containing added sugar, refined grains, trans fats, or hydrogenated oils are limited as these can increase inflammation in the body. An anti-inflammatory diet may also exclude foods to which you have an intolerance or sensitivity.

Arguably, the most popular and most heavily researched anti-inflammatory diet is the Mediterranean diet. Over 50 years ago, scientists began observing the eating habits in countries surrounding the Mediterranean, such as Italy and Greece, compared to that of the United States. Researchers found that the Mediterranean lifestyle was associated with a reduced risk of chronic diseases. While specific foods may vary depending on the region, the emphasis is always on eating *whole, minimally processed foods and avoiding added sugar, refined grains, trans fats, and hydrogenated oils in an effort to reduce chronic inflammation.* Chronic inflammation is considered a major contributor to cardiovascular disease, inflammatory bowel disease, diabetes, rheumatoid arthritis, Alzheimer's disease, and certain cancers.

# FOODS TO PRIORITIZE FOR PERFORMANCE AND ANTI-INFLAMMATORY BENEFITS

The recipes in this book use foods that help combat excess inflammation and free radicals to improve athletic performance and overall health. Here's a breakdown of the most common foods you'll find in the recipes.

**Avocados.** Rich in monounsaturated fats, vitamin E, vitamin C, and fiber, these fruits come with strong anti-inflammatory benefits. Try my Avocado Mousse (see page 211), Anti-Inflammatory Salad (see page 106), or Vegan Buddha Bowls (see page 121), just a few of the many recipes in this book featuring avocado.

**Beets and beet juice.** Drinking beet juice has been shown to help improve stamina, shorten recovery time between training sessions, and improve blood pressure levels. The nitrates naturally found in beets help increase blood flow, allowing for more oxygen to be delivered to your muscles. For maximum benefit, drink beet juice or my Berry-Beet Smoothie (see page 74) 30 minutes before your workout. (You may see supplements that say "beetroot" powder. That's a different name for beets!)

**Berries.** Research shows that athletes who consume berries prior to and after prolonged exercise experience less inflammation and oxidative stress. Berries contain several antioxidants, including anthocyanin, vitamin C, and resveratrol. Add a variety to your diet, such as blueberries, strawberries, raspberries, and blackberries. A few of the many berry-heavy recipes in this book are the Anti-Inflammatory Salad (see page 106), Gut Health Berry Smoothie (see page 77), Basic Overnight Oats (see page 85), Chia Pudding (see page 98), and Frozen Berry Yogurt Bites (see page 212).

**Cherries.** Cherries are very rich in antioxidants. Research has shown concentrated cherry juice to be beneficial in reducing inflammation. Drink it 30 minutes after strenuous exercise either plain or as part of a smoothie to help fight inflammation.

**Citrus fruits.** Rich in fiber, flavonoids, and vitamin C, citrus fruits can help fight inflammation and protect your immune system. Add oranges, lemons, limes, and grapefruits to smoothies, as part of your breakfast or snack, or on top of a salad. Try my Citrus Antioxidant Smoothie (see page 78) for a quick and refreshing breakfast.

**Cold-water fish.** Fish oil is the best source of omega-3 fatty acids, and eating seafood is your best option. When compared to meat, most fish contain around the same amount of protein but significantly more omega-3 fatty acids and less saturated fat. Fish also provides iron and vitamin B12. Choose cold-water fish (since the fat that protects the fish from the cold water is loaded with omega-3s), and the fattier the better. Salmon, albacore tuna, Atlantic mackerel, and sardines are just a few choices to incorporate into your diet regularly. If you're new to cooking fish, start by trying my Simple Baked Salmon (see page 144) or One-Pan Salmon and Roasted Vegetables (see page 145).

**Dark chocolate.** Dark chocolate is rich in magnesium and a type of antioxidant known as flavanols. Choose 70 percent or higher dark chocolate for the highest flavanol content. Try my easy Dark Chocolate Nut Clusters (see page 208) or No-Bake Brownies (see page 205).

**Egg yolks.** Egg yolks are rich in vitamins A and C and the antioxidants lutein and zeaxanthin. Although egg white omelets are often mistaken for being a healthier option, it's actually the yolks you want. You miss out on all the most important nutrients in an egg by eating only the whites! You can get your fill of egg yolks in my Farmers' Market Egg Casserole (see page 90) or Pressure Cooker Frittata (see page 100).

**Extra-virgin olive oil (EVOO).** EVOO is an excellent source of monounsaturated fats and antioxidants, but it should be used only for cooking at temperatures below 400°F because it has a low smoke point. You probably already know that EVOO makes an excellent addition to pasta dishes, but it's also my go-to for making dressings and sauces, such as Cilantro-Lime Vinaigrette (see page 105), Chimichurri Sauce (see page 129), and Basil Pesto (see page 147).

**Nuts and seeds.** Flaxseed and chia seeds are rich in fiber, vitamin E, and omega-3 fatty acids. The form of omega-3s these seeds contain is alpha-linolenic acid (ALA), which is an excellent option for vegans or vegetarians who do not eat fish. Walnuts also contain ALA. When it comes to nuts and nut butters, aim for a variety. Each nut has a unique nutrient content, so by occasionally switching among all different kinds, you'll consume a wider variety of nutrients. For example, almonds are high in monounsaturated fats and vitamin E, peanuts are high in protein, cashews are high in magnesium, and brazil nuts are one of the best food sources of selenium. For athletes with nut allergies, sunflower seeds (and sunflower seed butter) and pumpkin seeds are good sources of vitamin E and healthy fats.

**Spices and herbs.** Many spices contain strong anti-inflammatory compounds. Two of the most popular are turmeric and ginger. A recent study also found that curcumin, a compound in turmeric, has a similar efficacy to diclofenac, a nonsteroidal anti-inflammatory drug (NSAID). Curcumin also demonstrated better tolerance among patients with knee osteoarthritis. Add a pinch of different spices and herbs to smoothies or sprinkle them in your meals to boost flavor and nutrient content.

**Vegetables.** Rich in vitamins, minerals, and antioxidants, vegetables may be the most essential food in fighting inflammation and protecting your immune system. Some of the richest sources that I recommend eating regularly include bell peppers, onions, beets, mushrooms, broccoli, sweet potatoes, and leafy greens like kale, spinach, and collards. Learn how to make Baked Sweet Potatoes and Steamed Collard Greens on page 179.

**Whole grains and legumes.** Whole grains and legumes contain fiber, antioxidants, and protein. Whole grains such as quinoa, rice, oats, buckwheat, millet, and barley are just a few of the many grain options. I recommend incorporating a variety of rice into your diet—brown, black (aka "forbidden"), jade pearl, jasmine, and wild rice—as these all vary in flavor, texture, and nutrient content. Sprouted grains and beans are also an excellent option, as the sprouting process can increase the bioavailability of the nutrients. Sprouted grains and legumes can also be easier for some people to digest. You can buy sprouted grain bread, sprouted beans, sprouted quinoa, and sprouted green lentils at Trader Joe's, Whole Foods Market, and some well-stocked grocery stores.

It's evident that incorporating a variety of these plant foods mentioned above—vegetables, fruits, whole grains, legumes, nuts, and seeds—on a daily basis has significant health benefits. Unfortunately, consumption of plant foods, especially fruits and vegetables, in the United States is far below the recommended levels. According to the Centers for Disease Control, only 9 percent of American adults meet the recommended daily vegetable intakes (2 to 3 cups per day) and only 12 percent meet the recommended fruit intake (1.5 to 2 cups per day). I recommend that you first determine how many servings of fruits and vegetables you usually eat per day, then begin using the recipes in this book to increase your intakes. If you find that you're currently averaging only 1 cup of vegetables per day, challenge yourself to see if you can increase this by 1 or even 2 cups. If you find yourself eating only one type of nut, whole grain, or fruit, make a point to branch out and try a new food from this book each week. You might discover a new food, or several, that you never thought you'd enjoy.

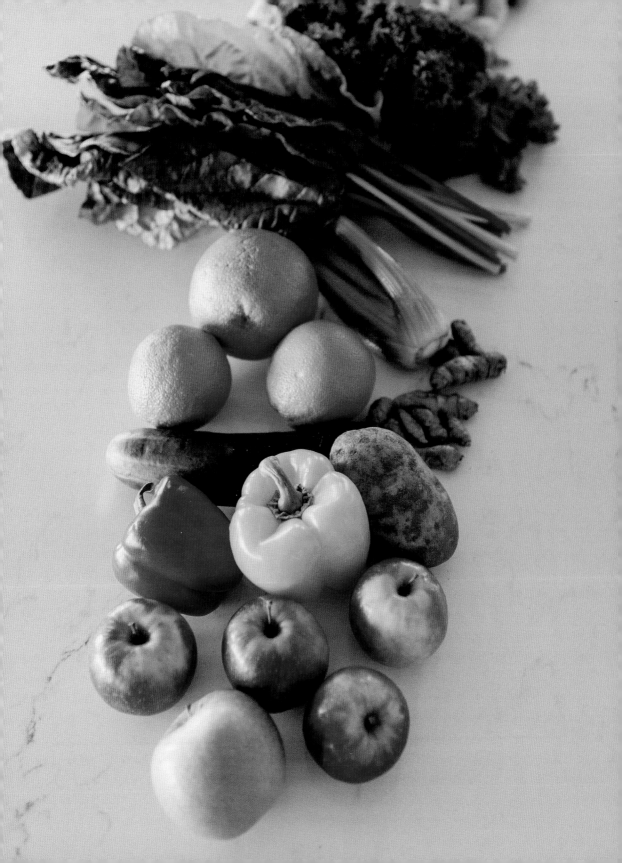

# PERFORMANCE NUTRITION MYTHS

**MYTH:**
Fruit has too much sugar.

**Fact:** Whole fruits contain an abundance of antioxidants, vitamins, minerals, and fiber. Eat whole fruits instead of drinking fruit juice, and if you're looking to reduce your sugar intake, try forgoing packaged bars, snack foods, and cereal—the things that don't grow on trees!

**MYTH:**
Coconut water alone can replace sports drinks.

**Fact:** While coconut water does provide fluid and carbohydrates during your workout, the huge drawback for athletes is the lack of sodium. You primarily lose sodium—not potassium—in your sweat. So relying solely on coconut water as your form of electrolyte replenishment could completely backfire. If you're looking for an alternative to traditional sports drinks, try my Homemade Sports Drinks (see page 186).

**MYTH:**
Vegan/vegetarian athletes can't get enough protein to support training.

**Fact:** Vegan and vegetarian athletes definitely can meet their protein needs, as long as they consume a variety of plant-based foods containing protein such as tofu, tempeh, edamame, lentils, beans, nuts, seeds, and peas. Supplementing with a plant-based protein powder that contains a blend of different sources may also help you meet your daily protein needs. For vegetarians who eat eggs or dairy, incorporating these two will increase total protein intake as well.

**MYTH:**
A keto diet is best for optimal performance.

**Fact:** There is no evidence that a keto diet improves athletic performance more than a diet higher in carbohydrates. It's actually shown to do quite the opposite, impairing both training intensity and duration in athletes performing at high intensities. An abundance of research shows the benefits carbohydrates have on improving both anaerobic and aerobic performance.

**MYTH:**
Egg yolks are unhealthy; you should only eat the egg whites.

**Fact:** Egg yolks are loaded with nutrition—they're rich in vitamins A and D, fatty acids, and antioxidants like lutein and zeaxanthin. For the most nutrition, eat the whole egg!

---

**MYTH:**
The more protein you eat, the more muscle you'll gain.

**Fact:** You won't gain muscle just by eating excessive amounts of protein. Muscle growth requires strength training and consuming adequate calories from all three macronutrient groups (carbohydrates, protein, and fat). If you consume large amounts of protein but are in a calorie deficit with insufficient carbohydrates and fats, your body will use protein stores for energy, making it even more difficult to gain muscle.

---

**MYTH:**
To lose weight, a low-carb diet is best.

**Fact:** When researchers compare low-carb diets to low-fat diets, they find no long-term differences as far as weight loss goes. If your goal is to lose weight, there must be a calorie deficit—regardless of whether that comes from small amounts of fat or carbohydrates, or both.

---

**MYTH:**
You shouldn't eat after 7:00 p.m. (or late at night).

**Fact:** It doesn't matter what *time* you're eating as much as *what* and *how much* you're eating throughout the entire day. Your body won't automatically start turning everything you eat into "fat" just because it's late at night. When late-night snacking takes a turn toward mindlessly munching on potato chips and pastries or drinking alcohol, then yes, this could absolutely lead to unwanted fat gain.

---

**MYTH:**
Gluten causes inflammation.

**Fact:** Unless you have diagnosed celiac disease or a gluten sensitivity, a gluten-free diet is often unnecessary and isn't shown to reduce inflammation or improve athletic performance. Removing all grains from your diet can also result in too little fiber intake.

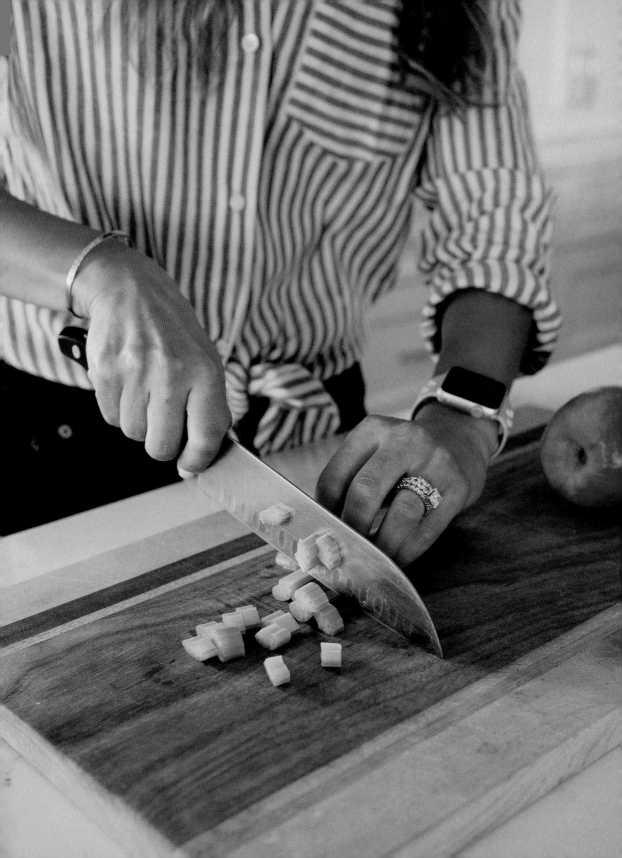

# PART TWO

## MEAL PLANNING AND KITCHEN BASICS

# CHAPTER THREE
## MEAL PREP AND PLANNING

"Meal prep" refers to scheduling time to prepare several meals at once and dividing them into individual portions so they're ready for you to reheat or grab-and-go. For example, you might set aside a couple of hours on Sunday doing meal prep for Monday through Wednesday, then do the other half midweek. (While you can certainly cook all of your week's meals on Sunday, I don't recommend it. By the middle of the week, the remainder of your meals won't be very appetizing. Especially if your meals contain animal protein, you should eat them within three or four days.) Meal prepping also means that you plan ahead for quick meals throughout the week so you have all the necessary ingredients on hand to save time later.

Meal prepping has become popular as a way to help save both time and money, which makes it particularly beneficial to high-performance athletes. If you plan out exactly what you're going to cook each week, you purchase accordingly and prevent waste. This also helps you avoid having to make several trips to the grocery store during the week. While it may seem time-consuming on the day you're preparing the meals, that extra hour or two goes a long way when it then takes only a few minutes to reheat already prepared meals throughout the week. Furthermore, having meals ready ahead of time may prevent you from stopping for fast food at the last minute on the way home.

For those wanting to make changes to body composition, meal prepping allows you to better control portion size. In order to make your meals last several days, you'll need to divide the food accordingly into separate containers. This helps you to portion out meals based on your goals, whether you're looking to gain, lose, or maintain weight.

Here are five tips to help you master meal prepping:

**1. Start simple.** Begin with simple meals that are easy for you to make and that you enjoy and know you'll look forward to eating as leftovers. The first recipes that come to my mind are Sweet Potato and Turkey Chili (see page 113) and Lentil Chili (see page 114). My chili recipes are very simple, take little time to prepare, and taste great as leftovers. One batch of either makes five or six servings, so you'll be set for many days of meals. If you don't want to eat the same thing every day, Lentil Tacos (see page 126) are a great choice. The lentil mixture that serves as the base of the tacos can be repurposed later in the week for a taco salad or served with rice and vegetables for a grain bowl. This allows for a bit more versatility.

**2. Take advantage of shortcuts.** There's no question that chopping, dicing, and mincing can take quite a bit of time, which can make you dread meal prep. But by purchasing jars of minced garlic, frozen chopped onions, canned beans, and precooked rice, you can significantly cut your prepping time.

**3. Cook in batches.** Whether you're cooking for a family of five or just for yourself, batch cooking can be a real time-saver. Batch cooking simply means doubling or even tripling a recipe to allow for ample leftovers that you can either eat later in the week or freeze for another day some weeks or months down the road. It takes less time and effort to prepare a double batch of some recipes—my Mexican-Inspired Chicken Casserole (see page 171) is a great candidate—than to prepare a single batch of the same recipe on two different nights.

**4. Write it down.** When you create your weekly meal plan, take the time to write down exactly what you'll need for each recipe. Check your pantry and fridge, then make your shopping list before heading to the store. Also be sure to take a look at your training schedule to determine the best days and times to do your meal prep. A little planning will help save you time and make meal prepping so much easier.

**5. Break it down into four simple categories.** You can either prep complete meals, soups, and casseroles using set recipes or use the simple meal prep formula I've created, shown below. Build your meals by choosing one from **each** of the categories—these are just a few of many examples.

| VEGETABLES | PROTEIN | HEALTHY FATS | CARBOHYDRATES |
|---|---|---|---|
| Leafy greens (collard greens, spinach, kale) | Eggs | Avocado | Oats |
| | Fish | Olives | Rice |
| Brussels sprouts | Chicken | Olive oil | Quinoa |
| Broccoli | Turkey | Avocado oil | Whole-grain pasta |
| Green beans | Tofu | Nuts | |
| Cauliflower | Tempeh | Nut butters | Whole-grain bread |
| Bok choy | Beans and legumes (also provide carbohydrates) | Seeds | Potatoes |
| Cabbage | | | Sweet potatoes |
| Celery | | | |
| Squash | | | |

Bonus: How many different kinds of vegetables can you incorporate into your diet each week? For example, if you notice you're eating only broccoli and carrots every week, try adding at least one or two new vegetables each week, especially focusing on a rainbow of different colors so you can get a variety of nutrients—try beets, bell peppers, and cauliflower.

The struggle I often see with athletes getting started with meal prepping is that they think it has to be "all or nothing." Don't feel obligated to prep every single meal and snack you plan to eat during the day. Instead, take note of the meals that you struggle with most. Are you constantly rushed in the mornings and running out of time for breakfast? It may be most beneficial for you to at least prep your breakfast so you can simply grab it as you head out the door. Try these recipes: Basic Overnight Oats (see page 85), Morning Muesli (see page 86), Farmers' Market Egg Casserole (see page 90), and Baked Oatmeal Casserole (see page 94). If you prefer a performance snack before an early morning workout, you might want to make my 3-Ingredient Energy Bars (see page 187) to eat along with a piece of fruit instead of a full breakfast.

Are you coming home late at night exhausted after a day of training or practice? Do you often rely on takeout for dinner because you're too tired to start cooking dinner from scratch? In that case, it might be most beneficial for you to focus on meal prepping your dinners. If you're someone who finds leftovers unappealing, you could at least prep a little in advance by taking advantage of shortcuts, such as buying prechopped items or chopping and storing your own vegetables a day in advance. You might also find the recipes labeled in this cookbook as "30 Minutes or Less" to be your favorites on busy nights.

# SAMPLE MEAL PLANS

To help simplify your meal planning even more, I've included three sample meal plans and corresponding lists of the ingredients you'll need: one for weight management, one for weight gain, and another for vegan or vegetarian athletes. The recipes for each meal plan were chosen because they make excellent leftovers, which will help reduce your time in the kitchen while still providing plenty of variety so you never get bored eating the same things. The lists may look long at first, but if you follow my kitchen staples guidance (see page 60), you'll only need to grab a few things each week to make your meals. The main difference between the weight management and weight gain meals is the portion size, so regardless of your goal, you can swap any of the recipes in these meal plans with another in this book. Keep in mind that everyone has their own individual energy needs (see page 21), so feel free to adjust the portion sizes suggested here or make other modifications to best fit your lifestyle.

▶ Weight management meal plan | page 44

▶ Weight gain meal plan | page 48

▶ Vegetarian/Vegan meal plan | page 52

# WEIGHT MANAGEMENT MEAL PLAN

|  | MON | TUE | WED |
|---|---|---|---|
| **Breakfast** | 1 serving Baked Oatmeal Casserole (page 94) | 1 serving Baked Oatmeal Casserole | 1 serving Baked Oatmeal Casserole |
| **Morning Snack** | 1 Citrus Antioxidant Smoothie (page 78) | 1 serving Parmesan-Roasted Edamame (page 190) | 1 Simple Green Smoothie (page 74) |
| **Lunch** | 1 serving Anti-Inflammatory Salad with Honey-Lemon Vinaigrette (page 106) | 1 serving Anti-Inflammatory Salad with Honey-Lemon Vinaigrette | 1 serving Shredded Salsa Chicken Burrito Bowls (page 117) |
| **Dinner** | 1 serving Shrimp and Broccoli Stir-Fry (page 148) | 1 serving Turkey Bolognese (page 151) with zucchini noodles | 1 serving Simple Baked Salmon (page 144) with ½ cup quinoa and 1 cup vegetables |
| **Late-Night Snack** | ½ cup Frozen Berry Yogurt Bites (page 212) | 1 No-Bake Brownie (page 205) | 2 Almond Flour Chocolate Chip Cookies (page 201) |

| THU | FRI | SAT | SUN |
| --- | --- | --- | --- |
| 1 Coffee and Cacao Smoothie (page 81) | 1 serving Farmers' Market Egg Casserole (page 90) | 1 serving Farmers' Market Egg Casserole | 1 Breakfast Parfait (page 93), or 1 serving Farmers' Market Egg Casserole |
| 1 serving Chia Pudding (page 98) | 1 Peppermint-Cacao Green Smoothie (page 81) | 1 serving Parmesan-Roasted Edamame | 1 serving Chia Pudding |
| 1 serving Shredded Salsa Chicken Burrito Bowls | 1 serving Sweet Potato and Turkey Chili | 1 serving Sweet Potato and Turkey Chili, or 1 serving Shredded Salsa Chicken Burrito Bowls | 1 serving Honey-Garlic Chicken (page 172) |
| 1 serving Sweet Potato and Turkey Chili (page 113) | 1 serving Simple Baked Salmon with ½ cup quinoa and 1 cup vegetables | 1 serving One-Pan Chicken and Veggie Dinner (page 181) | 2 slices Buffalo Chicken Pizza (page 167) with a mixed-greens side salad |
| ½ cup Frozen Berry Yogurt Bites | 1 No-Bake Brownie | 2 Almond Flour Chocolate Chip Cookies | ½ cup Frozen Berry Yogurt Bites |

# WEIGHT MANAGEMENT: WHAT YOU'LL NEED

### SPICES AND SEASONINGS

arrowroot or cornstarch

baking soda

black pepper

buffalo sauce, such as
The New Primal

cacao nibs, raw  *optional*

cacao powder

cayenne pepper

chili powder

cinnamon, ground

cumin, ground

garlic powder

honey

maple syrup, pure

oil, avocado

oil, coconut

oil, extra-virgin olive

oil, toasted sesame

oregano, dried

paprika, smoked

parsley, dried

peppermint extract

salt

seasoning blend of choice

tamari

turmeric, ground

vanilla extract

vinegar, apple cider

vinegar, white balsamic

### FLOURS, GRAINS, SEEDS, AND NUTS

almond butter, creamy
*2 tablespoons*

almonds, sliced  *⅓ cup*

almonds, whole  *¼ cup*

chia seeds  *¼ cup*

chickpea crumbs  *½ cup*

flour, almond  *2 cups*

oats, old-fashioned
rolled  *6 cups*

peanut butter,
creamy  *⅓ cup*

quinoa  *½–¾ cup*

rice, brown  *2 cups*

sesame seeds  *optional*

walnuts, chopped  *2 cups*

### FRESH PRODUCE AND HERBS

apple, green  *1*

apple of choice  *1*

avocado  *2 or 3*

banana  *6*

basil, small bunch  *1*

bell pepper, green  *2*

blueberries  *4 cups*

broccoli florets, fresh or
frozen  *1 cup*

brussels sprouts  *2 cups/
about 16 sprouts*

celery stalk  *2*

cucumber  *1*

dates, Medjool  *2 cups*

edamame, shelled, fresh
or frozen  *1 (10-ounce)
package*

fruit of choice,
chopped  *1 cup*

garlic head  *1*

ginger  *1 (2-inch) piece*

greens, mixed
*1 (5-ounce) package*

kale, large bunch  *1 or 2*

lemon  *2*

mushrooms of
choice  *½ cup*

onion, red  *1*

onion, white  *3*

orange  *1*

parsley, small
bunch  *optional*

potato, medium  *3*

potato, petite rainbow
*2 pounds*

romaine lettuce,
shredded  *1 (10-ounce)
bag*

spinach  *1½–2 pounds*

sweet potato, large  *1*

thyme, small bunch  *1*

tomato  *1 or 2*

vegetables of
choice  *2 cups*

zucchini, large  *3*

## PREPARED AND PACKAGED FOODS

beans, black  *2 (15-ounce)
cans*

broth, low-sodium
chicken  *3 cups*

chocolate bar, 72% dark  *1*

chocolate chips,
dark  *½ cup*

coconut milk,
unsweetened plain
*1 tablespoon; optional*

coconut water  *1 cup*

coffee, cold-brewed
*8 ounces*

dried fruit of
choice  *¼ cup; optional*

guacamole  *optional*

marinara sauce  *⅓ cup*

pizza crust, 12-inch
whole-wheat  *1*

salsa  *1 (15-ounce) jar*

shredded coconut,
unsweetened  *½ cup*

tomatoes, crushed
*2 (28-ounce) cans*

## REFRIGERATOR AND FREEZER ITEMS

cheese of choice,
shredded  *⅓ cup*

mango chunks,
frozen  *1 cup*

mozzarella cheese,
shredded  *½ cup*

nondairy milk,
unsweetened  *3¾ cups*

nondairy milk,
unsweetened
vanilla  *3½ cups*

parmesan cheese,
grated  *⅓ cup*

yogurt, plain Greek
*2 (16-ounce) containers*

## PROTEINS

chicken breasts, boneless,
skinless  *3½ pounds*

eggs, large  *13*

protein powder of
choice  *1 scoop*

salmon, wild-caught
*1 pound*

shrimp  *8 ounces*

turkey, lean ground
*2½ pounds*

# WEIGHT GAIN MEAL PLAN

| | MON | TUE | WED |
|---|---|---|---|
| **Breakfast** | 2 servings Baked Oatmeal Casserole (page 94) with 2–3 scrambled eggs | 2 servings Baked Oatmeal Casserole with 2–3 scrambled eggs | 1 Chocolate-Banana Smoothie made with ½ cup oats, plus 2–3 eggs |
| **Morning Snack** | 1 Chocolate-Banana Smoothie (page 78) made with ½ cup oats | 1 Tropical Green Smoothie (page 77) made with 1 scoop protein powder and avocado | 1 Breakfast Parfait (page 93) |
| **Lunch** | 2 servings Mexican-Inspired Chicken Casserole (page 171) | 2 servings Mexican-Inspired Chicken Casserole | 2 servings Shredded Salsa Chicken Burrito Bowls (page 117) with 1½ cups brown rice |
| **Afternoon Snack** | 6 Post-Workout Recovery Bites (page 184) or 3-Ingredient Energy Bars (page 187) | 1 serving Avocado Toast with Hard-Boiled Eggs (page 195) | 6 Post-Workout Recovery Bites or 3-Ingredient Energy Bars |
| **Dinner** | 2 servings Thai Peanut Chicken (page 164) with 1½ cups brown rice | 2 servings Turkey Bolognese (page 151) with 1 cup zucchini and 2 cups whole-grain spaghetti | 2 servings Simple Baked Salmon (page 144) with 1 cup quinoa and 1 cup vegetables |
| **Late-Night Snack** | 1 Simple Green Smoothie (page 74) or 1 Chocolate-Banana Smoothie (optional; add ½ cup oats for additional calories) | | |

| THU | FRI | SAT | SUN |
| --- | --- | --- | --- |
| 2 servings Morning Muesli (page 86) | 2 servings Sweet Potato and Black Bean Hash (page 89) with 3 over easy eggs | 2 servings Farmers' Market Egg Casserole (page 90) with 2 slices whole-grain bread and ½ avocado | 2 servings Farmers' Market Egg Casserole with 2 slices whole-grain bread and ½ avocado |
| 1 serving Avocado Toast with Hard-Boiled Eggs | ¾–1 cup Endurance Trail Mix (page 190) | 6 Post-Workout Recovery Bites or 3-Ingredient Energy Bars | 6 Post-Workout Recovery Bites or 3-Ingredient Energy Bars |
| 2 servings Shredded Salsa Chicken Burrito Bowls | 2 servings Sweet Potato and Turkey Chili with ½ avocado | 2 servings Sweet Potato and Turkey Chili, Shredded Salsa Chicken Burrito Bowls, or One-Pan Chicken and Veggie Dinner with 1½ cups brown rice and at least ½ avocado | 2 servings Slow or Instant Turkey Meatballs (page 153) with 1½ cups whole-grain pasta and 1 cup vegetables |
| 1 Tropical Green Smoothie made with 1 scoop protein powder and avocado | 6 Post-Workout Recovery Bites or 3-Ingredient Energy Bars | 1 Tropical Green Smoothie with 1 scoop protein powder and avocado | 1 Chocolate-Banana Smoothie made with ½ cup oats |
| 2 servings Sweet Potato and Turkey Chili (page 113) with ½ avocado | 2 servings One-Pan Chicken and Veggie Dinner (page 181) with 1½ cups brown rice | 4–5 slices Buffalo Chicken Pizza (page 167) with a mixed-greens side salad with olive oil | 2 servings Whole-Grain Pesto Fusilli with Scallops (page 147) |

1 Simple Green Smoothie or 1 Chocolate-Banana Smoothie

# WEIGHT GAIN: WHAT YOU'LL NEED

### SPICES AND SEASONINGS

basil, dried

black pepper

buffalo sauce, such as The New Primal

cacao powder

cayenne pepper

chile paste

chili powder

cinnamon, ground

coriander, ground

cumin, ground

cumin seeds

garlic powder

honey

maple syrup, pure

oil, avocado

oil, coconut

oil, extra-virgin olive

oil, toasted sesame

oregano, dried

paprika, smoked

paprika, sweet

parsley, dried

red pepper flakes

salt

seasoning blend of choice

tamari

vanilla extract

vinegar, rice

vinegar, white balsamic

### FLOURS, GRAINS, SEEDS, AND NUTS

almonds, sliced  *1 cup*

almonds, whole  *1 cup*

bread, sprouted-grain loaf  *1*

bread, whole-grain loaf  *1*

breadcrumbs, whole-wheat  *¼ cup*

cashews  *1 cup*

cereal of choice  *2 cups*

chia seeds  *1 tablespoon*

fusilli, whole-grain  *1 (16-ounce) package*

granola  *½ cup*

oats, rolled old-fashioned  *1 (42-ounce) package*

peanut butter, creamy  *2 (16-ounce) jars*

peanuts  *½ cup*

pine nuts  *¼ cup*

pumpkin seeds  *½ cup*

quinoa  *1 cup*

rice, brown  *2 (1-pound) bags*

spaghetti, whole-grain  *1 (16-ounce) package*

sunflower seeds  *½ cup*

walnuts, chopped  *1 cup*

wheat flakes  *1 cup*

### FRESH PRODUCE AND HERBS

apple, green  *5*

avocado  *9*

banana  *8*

basil, large bunch  *2*

bell pepper, green  *3*

berries of choice  *1 cup*

broccoli florets  *2 cups*

brussels sprouts  *1 cup*

cilantro, small bunch  *1*

dates  *½ cup*

fruit of choice, chopped  *1 cup*

garlic head  *1–2*

greens, mixed  *1 (5-ounce) package*

kale  *1½–2 pounds*

lemon  *2*

lime  *1*

mushrooms of choice
½ cup

onion, red  1

onion, white  5

parsley, small bunch  1

potato, medium  3

potato, petite rainbow
2 pounds

romaine lettuce,
shredded  1 (10-ounce)
bag

scallions, small bunch  1

spinach  1 pound

sweet potato, large  3

thyme, small bunch  1

tomato  1 or 2

tomato, cherry  ½ cup

vegetables of choice
1 cup

zucchini, large  4

## PREPARED AND PACKAGED FOODS

beans, black  4 (15-ounce)
cans

broth, low-sodium
chicken  3 cups

dried fruit of choice
¼ cup; optional

guacamole  optional

marinara sauce
2 (25-ounce) jars

pizza crust, 12-inch
whole-wheat  1

raisins  ½ cup

salsa  1 (15-ounce) jar

shredded coconut,
unsweetened  ½ cup

tomatoes, crushed
2 (28-ounce) cans

tomatoes, diced fire-
roasted  1 (14.5-ounce)
can

## REFRIGERATOR AND FREEZER ITEMS

cheddar cheese,
shredded  ½ cup

cheese of choice,
shredded  ⅓ cup

mango chunks, frozen
1½ cups

mozzarella cheese,
shredded  1 cup

nondairy milk,
unsweetened  13¾ cups

parmesan cheese,
grated  ¾ cup

pineapple chunks,
frozen  1½ cups

vegetables, frozen mixed
stir-fry  2 cups

yogurt, plain Greek
3 (16-ounce) containers

yogurt, whole-milk  1 cup

## PROTEINS

chicken breasts, boneless,
skinless  5½ pounds

eggs, large  3 dozen

protein powder of
choice  1 large container

salmon, wild-caught
1 pound

scallops  1 pound

turkey, ground  3¾ pounds

# VEGETARIAN/VEGAN MEAL PLAN

|  | MON | TUE | WED |
|---|---|---|---|
| **Breakfast** | 1 serving Basic Overnight Oats (page 85) | 1 serving Sweet Potato and Black Bean Hash (page 89) | 1 serving No-Sugar-Added Acai Bowl (page 101) |
| **Morning Snack** | 1 Citrus Antioxidant Smoothie (page 78) | 1 serving Cashew Queso (page 192) with plantain chips | 1 Simple Green Smoothie (page 74) |
| **Lunch** | 1 serving Anti-Inflammatory Salad with Honey-Lemon Vinaigrette (page 106) with ½ cup roasted chickpeas or 2 hard-boiled eggs | 1 serving Spicy Pad Thai with Tofu (page 139) | 1 serving Vegan Buddha Bowls (page 121) |
| **Dinner** | 1 serving Lentil Chili (page 114) with sliced avocado on top | 1 serving Lentil Tacos (page 126) | 1 serving Tofu Parmesan (page 135) |
| **Late-Night Snack** | ½ cup Frozen Berry Yogurt Bites (page 212) | 1 No-Bake Brownie (page 205) | 1 serving Avocado Mousse (page 211) |

| THU | FRI | SAT | SUN |
|---|---|---|---|
| 1 Coffee and Cacao Smoothie (page 81) | 1 serving Baked Oatmeal Casserole (page 94) | 1 serving Tofu Scramble (page 136) | 1 serving Baked Oatmeal Casserole or Tofu Scramble |
| 1 serving Chia Pudding (page 98) | 1 Peppermint-Cacao Green Smoothie (page 81) | 1 serving 3-Ingredient Energy Bars (page 187) | 1 serving Chia Pudding |
| 1 serving Waldorf Kale Salad with Yogurt Dressing with edamame (page 109) | 1 serving Ramen Bowls (page 118) | 1 serving Tempeh Bolognese | 1 serving Ramen Bowls or Tempeh Bolognese |
| 1 serving Chickpea-Lentil Curry (page 115) | 1 serving Tempeh Bolognese (page 140) | 1 serving Chimichurri Mushroom Tacos (page 128) | 1 serving Chimichurri Mushroom Tacos, Chickpea-Lentil Curry, or Lentil Tacos |
| 1 Dark Chocolate Nut Cluster (page 208) | 1 No-Bake Brownie | 1 serving Raw Cookie Dough (page 202) | ½ cup Frozen Berry Yogurt Bites |

# VEGETARIAN/VEGAN: WHAT YOU'LL NEED

### SPICES AND SEASONINGS

baking soda

basil, dried

black pepper

cacao nibs, raw *optional*

cacao powder

cayenne pepper

chile paste

chili powder

cinnamon, ground

cocoa powder, unsweetened

coriander, ground

cumin, ground

garlic powder

honey

maple syrup, pure

mustard

oil, avocado

oil, extra-virgin olive

oil, toasted sesame

onion powder

oregano, dried

paprika, smoked

paprika, sweet

parsley, dried

peppermint extract

red pepper flakes

salt

taco seasoning

tamari

tikka seasoning, such as Spicemode

turmeric, ground

vanilla extract

vinegar, apple cider

vinegar, red wine

vinegar, rice

### FLOURS, GRAINS, SEEDS, AND NUTS

almond butter, creamy *6 tablespoons*

almonds, sliced *½ cup*

almonds, whole *¾ cup*

breadcrumbs, whole-wheat *¼ cup*

brown rice noodles, ramen *1 (2.8-ounce) package*

cashews *1¾ cups*

chia seeds *⅓ cup*

nuts of choice *¼ cup; optional*

oats, rolled old-fashioned *3¾ cups*

pasta, whole-grain *8 ounces*

peanut butter, creamy *¾ cup*

pistachios *¼ cup*

quinoa *1 cup*

rice, basmati *1 cup*

rice noodles *1 (8-ounce) package*

sesame seeds *optional*

walnuts, chopped *2¾ cups*

whole grain of choice, cooked *1 cup*

### FRESH PRODUCE AND HERBS

apple, green *1*

apple of choice *2*

avocado *9*

banana *8*

bell pepper, red *1*

bell pepper, green *2*

blueberries *5 cups*

carrot, large *6*

celery stalk *6*

cilantro, large bunch *1*

cucumber *1*

dates, Medjool *4 cups*

garlic head *1–2*

ginger *1-inch piece*

grapes, halved *½ cup*

jalapeño  *1*

kale  *2 pounds*

leafy greens of choice,
chopped  *2 cups*

lemon  *1*

lime  *2*

mushrooms, cremini  *½ cup*

mushrooms, portobello  *3*

mushrooms, shiitake
*8–10*

onion, white  *4*

onion, yellow  *1*

orange  *1*

parsley, small bunch  *1*

raspberries  *1 cup; optional*

romaine lettuce,
shredded  *2 cups*

scallions, chopped
*optional*

spinach  *4 cups*

sweet potato, large  *4*

tomato  *3*

## PREPARED AND PACKAGED FOODS

beans, black  *2 (15-ounce)
cans*

broth, low-sodium
vegetable  *9 cups*

chickpeas  *3 (15-ounce)
cans*

chickpeas, roasted  *½ cup*

chocolate, dark  *3 ounces*

chocolate bar, 72% dark  *1*

chocolate chips, dairy-free
dark  *¾ cup*

coconut flakes,
unsweetened  *1 tablespoon*

coconut milk, full-fat
*1 (13.5-ounce) can*

coconut milk,
unsweetened plain
*1 tablespoon; optional*

coconut sugar
*2 teaspoons*

coconut water  *1 cup*

coffee, cold-brewed
*8 ounces*

cranberries, dried
*2 tablespoons*

dressing of choice

marinara sauce  *8 ounces*

nutritional yeast  *¾ cup*

plantain chips  *1 serving*

tomato sauce
*1 (15-ounce) can*

tomatoes, crushed
*1 (28-ounce) can*

tomatoes, diced
*1 (15-ounce) can*

tortillas, corn  *12*

tortillas, small flour  *8*

wine, dry red  *⅓ cup*

## REFRIGERATOR AND FREEZER ITEMS

acai berry puree, frozen
unsweetened
*1 (3.5-ounce) packet*

cheese of choice,
shredded  *optional*

goat cheese, crumbled
*½ cup*

hash browns, frozen  *2 cups*

mango chunks, frozen
*1¼ cup*

nondairy milk,
unsweetened  *4⅓ cups*

nondairy milk, unsweet-
ened vanilla  *5 cups*

parmesan cheese,
grated  *¼ cup*

yogurt, plain Greek  *½ cup*

## PROTEINS

eggs, large  *3*

lentils, cooked brown
*2 cups*

lentils, green  *1 cup*

protein powder of
choice  *1 scoop; optional*

tempeh  *1 (8-ounce)
package*

tofu, extra-firm
*4 (15-ounce) packages*

# CHAPTER FOUR

# COOKING BASICS

Often, the athletes I work with have no experience in the kitchen. The thought of shopping for ingredients and cooking meals on their own seems impossible to them. Add this anxiety to the fact that most athletes have demanding schedules and may need to travel for competition, and it can be daunting to even think about adding another task—cooking—to your daily routine.

But there's good news. You don't need to be a trained chef to cook delicious, nourishing meals, and you can absolutely make them with limited skills and space with the right preparation, tools, and recipes. I'm here to walk you through the basics. This chapter will make you feel more comfortable about stocking your kitchen and pantry, as well as understanding common cooking terms used in recipes. And for anyone feeling particularly uncertain about getting started, I've included a section of practical tips (see page 63).

# COOKING METHODS

Let's start by discussing the different oven and stovetop cooking methods you'll find in this book: baking, boiling, broiling, roasting, sautéing, and simmering. These are common cooking methods that you'll see in recipes everywhere. Here's a simple breakdown of each:

**Baking.** When you bake, you're surrounding the food with hot, dry air. Baking temperatures usually go up to 375°F; go any higher and you're roasting (see below). You'll often see 350°F as the required temperature in this cookbook. It does take a little while for your oven to reach this temperature, which is why the first step of many baking recipes tells you to preheat your oven. This means that you need to wait until your oven has reached the given temperature before you put anything in to start baking. Every oven is different, but it usually takes about 15 minutes for an oven to fully preheat. You can use this time to prep your ingredients.

**Boiling.** Recipes may instruct you to boil water, or may even mention bringing something to a "rolling boil." Boiling is done by filling a pot with water and setting it on a stovetop burner turned to high heat. When bubbles break the surface, that's when the water has reached a rolling boil. Now it's ready to be used for pasta, rice, eggs, and even vegetables. After adding food to the boiling water, turn down the heat and monitor it to prevent the water from boiling over. You can make water boil faster by putting a lid on the pot while it heats.

**Broiling.** Broiling chars and browns food similar to grilling, but it's done in an oven. With a grill, you cook food directly over the heat source; with an oven broiler, you cook under the heat source. Your oven's broiler may be at the top of your oven or in a drawer below it. Most modern ovens allow you to set the broiler to "high" or "low," and the level needed is usually specified in recipes. Be careful when broiling, as this high temperature can cause food to burn very quickly. Broiling is often called for at the very end of baking or roasting dishes to achieve a browned, crisp topping. You won't find any recipes that call for broiling in this cookbook, but now you know what the "broil" setting on your oven is for!

**Roasting.** Roasting is similar to baking in that it's done in an oven, but there are two important differences. First, roasting is done at higher temperatures than baking, usually above 400°F. Second, roasting is typically done uncovered; otherwise, the food would stew in its own juices instead of roast. Roasting also requires some form of fat to prevent the food from burning. It usually produces a crisp, brown exterior and a soft or moist interior.

**Sautéing.** When a recipe tells you to "sauté" something, typically vegetables, it means you cook them quickly in a small amount of oil. This is done in a skillet or sauté pan over medium to medium-high heat, and you use a spatula to help move the food around as it cooks, allowing for even cooking throughout. You first heat the oil in the pan before adding the vegetables or other ingredients. You can tell when the oil is hot enough when it slides easily in the pan and the surface appears to ripple or "shimmer."

**Simmering.** When a recipe mentions allowing a sauce to "simmer," it means the liquid should be barely bubbling, not at a rolling boil. To get from a rolling boil to simmering, simply turn the heat down from high to low or medium-low. You may need to adjust the heat to keep the liquid at a simmer.

# BASIC KNIFE TECHNIQUES

When reading through the recipes in this book, you'll find the words *chopped* and *minced*, referring mainly to vegetables and herbs. When you chop something, you simply cut it into small pieces, about ½ inch or so, but they don't need to be perfect. (In other cookbooks, you might see the word *diced*, which means to cut foods into neat cubes. That won't be required here!) If a food needs to be cut into smaller pieces—¼ or ⅛ inch—the recipe will specify *finely chopped*. And for garlic, you'll need to cut it up as small as you possibly can, which is what *minced* means. Or you might want to purchase a garlic press, which gets the job done much more quickly.

# KITCHEN STAPLES

A well-stocked pantry is essential for preparing nutritious meals. Here are the key ingredients you'll need to make most of the recipes in this cookbook.

## SPICE CABINET

Keep all spices tightly sealed and stored in a cool, dry place away from heat. If you own a spice rack, this should be stored far from your stovetop or windows with direct sunlight. The shelf life of spices varies depending on the type, and most have a "best by" date printed on the jar. If you notice that the freshness or flavor of a spice has dulled, it's probably time to toss it and get a new jar.

| | | |
|---|---|---|
| Black pepper | Dried parsley | Red pepper flakes |
| Cayenne pepper | Ground cinnamon | Smoked paprika |
| Chili powder | Ground cumin | Sweet paprika |
| Dried basil | Ground ginger | Table salt or sea salt |
| Dried oregano | Ground turmeric | |

## LEGUMES AND GRAINS

Whole grains, dried beans, and canned beans can all be stored at room temperature, ideally away from heat, moisture, and air. If you purchase dry grains or legumes from the bulk section of the supermarket, it's a good idea to transfer them to an airtight container to prolong shelf life.

| | | |
|---|---|---|
| Canned or dried lentils, black beans, chickpeas, and pinto beans | Old-fashioned rolled oats (certified gluten-free if necessary) | Rice (black, brown, jade pearl, jasmine, and wild) |
| Gluten-free grains (amaranth, buckwheat, millet, sorghum, and teff) | Quinoa | Whole-grain pasta |

## NUTS AND SEEDS

Keep nuts and seeds tightly sealed and store in a cool, dark place. To prolong freshness, store in a tightly sealed container in your fridge.

Almonds

Cashews

Chia seeds

Ground flaxseed

Nut butters (peanut butter, almond butter, and cashew butter)

Pistachios

Pumpkin seeds

Sunflower seeds

Walnuts

## OILS

Keep cooking oils tightly sealed and store in a cool, dark place. Exposure to heat, air, or light, especially with extra-virgin olive oil, can cause your oils to become rancid.

Avocado oil

Coconut oil

Extra-virgin olive oil

Toasted sesame oil

## VINEGARS, SWEETENERS, AND OTHER STAPLES

Vinegars should be stored in a cool, dry place, and have a shelf life of several years. Check the label for a "best by" date. To prolong the freshness of sweeteners such as maple syrup, refrigerate after opening. Honey does not need to be refrigerated and is actually best stored at room temperature, tightly sealed and away from direct sunlight.

Avocados (when cut, store in fridge)

Coconut sugar

Garlic

Lemons and limes (to prolong freshness, store in fridge)

Maple syrup (100 percent pure)

Nutritional yeast

Onions (when cut, store in fridge)

Raw honey

Tamari (gluten-free soy sauce)

Vegetable broth, chicken broth, or bone broth (refrigerate after opening)

Vinegar (apple cider, red wine, rice, white balsamic)

## BAKING STAPLES

Store flours in airtight containers, in a cool, dry place. Most flours should last about 3 months, or up to 6 months in the freezer.

Almond meal/flour

Baking powder

Baking soda

Brown rice flour

Vanilla extract

Whole-wheat flour

# ESSENTIAL TOOLS FOR YOUR KITCHEN

The following kitchen gadgets are my recommended must-haves to take your cooking to the next level. While you definitely don't need everything on this list, even just having a few of these items will help you cook the recipes in this book with ease.

**Baking sheet.** A baking sheet, also referred to as a sheet pan, is a flat rectangular metal pan used for baking and roasting. It has a small lip around the entire outer edge to keep food or liquid from rolling or running off the sides. For easier cleanup, I recommend lining your baking sheet with parchment paper.

**Baking pans and casserole dishes.** Casseroles are easy meals and make for excellent leftovers. All you need is a standard 9 × 13-inch baking pan, but you might also want a deep, round casserole dish with a lid and handles. You'll also find an 8-inch or 9-inch square baking pan useful for smaller recipes.

**Chef's knife and paring knife.** I firmly believe that every home cook should have one good-quality chef's knife and one paring knife. This makes slicing and chopping for meal prep so much easier.

**High-speed blender.** This can double as a food processor. I talk more about the benefits of having a high-speed blender in the chapter on smoothies (page 69).

**Pots and pans.** Essentials include a 2- or 3-quart saucepan, a 6- to 12-quart stockpot, and a 10- to 12-inch nonstick skillet. Saucepans are round pots with straight sides, a long handle, and a lid. They can be tall or shallow and are most often used in this cookbook to boil water for eggs, quinoa, or pasta. I also recommend having one large pot, sometimes called a stockpot, which should hold 6 to 12 quarts and include a lid. Skillets, which are shallower than saucepans and usually have curved sides, can be used to make just about any meal. You might also want to invest in a 10- to 14-inch sauté pan, which is similar to a skillet except that it has straighter, higher sides.

**Slow cooker and/or pressure cooker.** Whether you're constantly busy with practice, work, or class, nothing is more useful when it comes to meal prepping than a slow cooker (such as a Crock-Pot) or electric pressure cooker (such as an Instant Pot). These are handy for athletes living in hotels without full kitchens or in dorm-style apartments without ovens or stoves—or for anyone who wants a hands-off approach to cooking.

That's all the big stuff you need. Now for the small stuff, much of which you may already have:

| | | |
|---|---|---|
| Can opener | Spatula | Vegetable peeler |
| Measuring cup set | Strainer or colander | Whisk |
| Measuring spoon set | Two cutting boards (one | |
| Mixing bowls | for raw meat, one for | |
| | everything else) | |

There are also a few items I recommend that are not strictly necessary. These include a food processor, box grater, cast-iron skillet, 12-cup muffin tin, and 9 × 5-inch loaf pan. That's it—now you're ready to cook!

# ADVICE FOR THOSE WHO DON'T KNOW WHERE TO START

Starting a new routine can be challenging, and when it comes to cooking, it can be difficult to know where to even begin. Athletes in particular have other challenges to take into consideration, such as extremely limited time, busy schedules, and travel. If that sounds like you, here are some tips.

**If you have limited access to a full kitchen.** Are you in a dorm room with no oven or stove? Are you having to spend weeks at a time living in a place with no access to a kitchen? If this is the case, I recommend looking for the "No Kitchen" symbol throughout this cookbook. This symbol will direct you to recipes that do not require a stove or oven. These recipes can be made with either a slow cooker or pressure cooker, or just a microwave and fridge. If you have limited access to a kitchen or if using an oven and stove overwhelms you, I recommend starting with a slow cooker.

**If you have never cooked on your own.** If an athlete has never cooked on their own before, I usually have them start with my Shredded Salsa Chicken Burrito Bowls (see page 117) or Shredded Buffalo Chicken (see page 159), both of which can be made in a slow cooker or pressure cooker. You'll often be given two options for slow cooker recipes—cooking on high for 3 hours or on low for 5 to 6 hours. This is a great option depending on your schedule for the day. If you plan to prep the slow cooker recipe first thing in the morning, set it on low, and once you get home that evening your meal will be finished cooking and ready to eat.

**If you don't have much time.** Pressure cookers are growing in popularity because they cook food much faster than slow cookers. For example, instead of setting a slow cooker on low for 5 hours for my Shredded Buffalo Chicken recipe, you can prepare it in a pressure cooker on high pressure for 14 minutes. Athletes tend to be more intimidated by pressure cookers than slow cookers, typically because of the dial that's used to seal and release pressure. But it's really simple: Turn to seal before cooking, and turn to release after cooking—that's it. You want the dial to be in the sealing position to allow steam to fill the pressure cooker first, then you want to make sure all that steam is released after cooking but before removing the lid to avoid the steam hitting you in the face.

I recommend skimming through each recipe and folding down the page corners of the ones that sound most appealing to you to start. If you find yourself confused with a cooking term, go back to the cooking basics section on page 57.

# HOW TO USE THIS BOOK

I realize many of you reading this may be cooking for the very first time on your own, while others may have several years of experience cooking. Either way, my goal is to make you feel as comfortable and confident as possible in the kitchen.

Before you begin cooking, I always recommend you read through the entire recipe first. Then lay out all the ingredients you will need in advance, as well as all the necessary measuring and cooking utensils. If you're completely new to cooking, don't be afraid to use shortcuts at the beginning. I mentioned when I discussed meal prep and planning on page 40 that purchasing minced garlic, chopped onion, and even cooked rice can save you a lot of time if you have a very tight schedule. However, taking shortcuts like this is also a helpful strategy for beginners who may feel overwhelmed by too many steps in a recipe.

I truly believe you'll be pleasantly surprised by the simplicity of the steps and ingredient lists in these recipes. I've also provided cooking, serving, and performance tips along the way to provide even more guidance with these recipes.

I've also included labels in the book to help you find the recipes that suit your dietary restrictions and lifestyle quickly. These symbols will help you navigate through this cookbook.

| | |
|---|---|
| **DF** | These recipes are **dairy-free**. They do not contain milk, butter, cheese, or yogurt. |
| **GF** | These recipes are **gluten-free**. They do not contain any ingredients, such as wheat, that include gluten. Remember to always double-check product labels to make sure they are certified gluten-free. |
| **NF** | These recipes are **nut-free**. They do not contain peanuts or tree nuts (almonds, cashews, walnuts, etc.), but they may contain coconut. |
| **VEG/V** | These recipes are either **vegetarian** (VEG), which means they do not contain meat or fish, or **vegan** (V), which means they don't contain any animal products, including dairy, eggs, and honey. |
| **30** | These recipes can be made from start to finish in **30 minutes or less**. |
| **NK** | These recipes can be made with **limited kitchen space** or **no kitchen**. They do not require an oven or stove. Many use a slow cooker, a pressure cooker, or a microwave and fridge. This makes them great for athletes who travel. |
| **OP** | These recipes are made entirely in **one pot or pan**—talk about easy! In some cases the "pan" is just your bowl or blender jar, but the point is that you'll have only one cooking vessel to wash! |

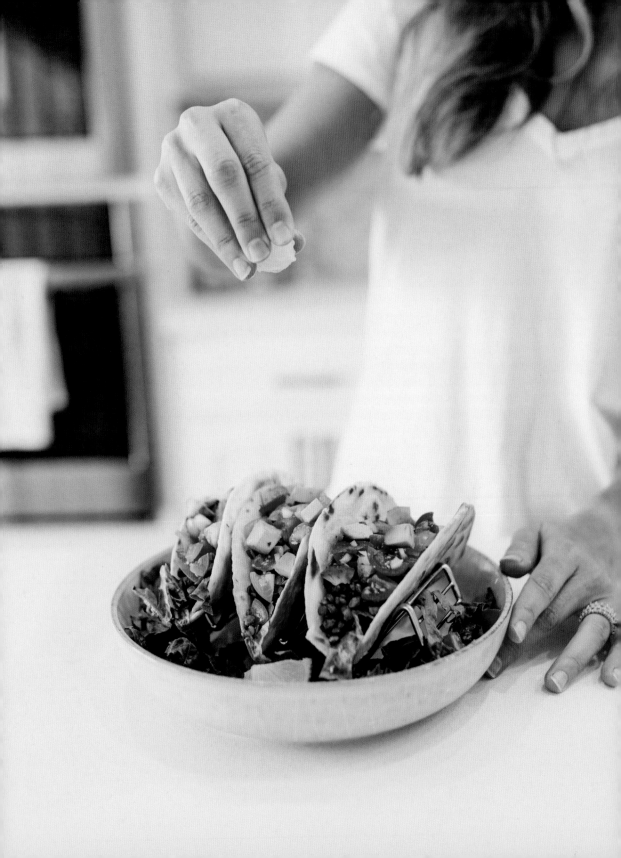

# PART THREE

# RECIPES

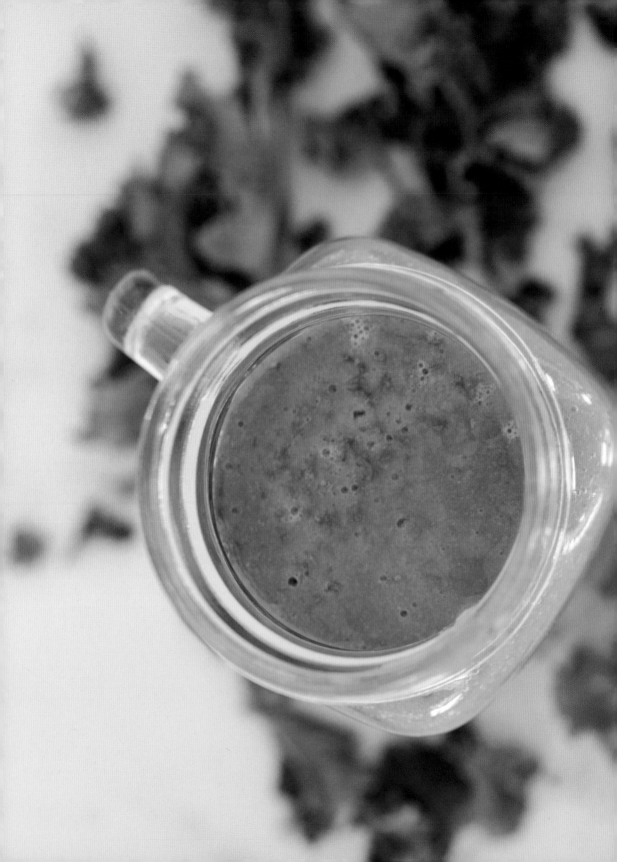

# CHAPTER FIVE

# THE PERFECT SMOOTHIE

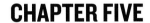

**S**moothies make delicious grab-and-go breakfasts or snacks and are a great way to get loads of nutrition with little time and effort. They are the perfect addition to your meal plan, whether you are looking to lose, maintain, or gain weight, while increasing your intake of antioxidant-rich fruits and vegetables. If you're someone who has a hard time eating breakfast, you might find a smoothie to be less daunting first thing in the morning than sitting down to a plate of food. Likewise, smoothies provide a great solution for athletes who find it difficult to tolerate solid foods post-workout.

Smoothies tend to get a bad rap because of the sugar content found in those sold at restaurants or popular smoothie chains. These smoothies are often made with fruit juice, frozen yogurt, ice cream, agave, or other high-sugar ingredients that make them more like dessert. Making your own smoothies at home will not only save you money but also allow you to add fiber, protein, and fats that help keep you full. If you're used to ultrasweet smoothies made with ice cream or frozen yogurt, the smoothie recipes in this chapter may not taste very sweet to you. One way you can work your way toward enjoying vegetable and fruit smoothies more is by adding just a teaspoon or two of honey and then slowly decreasing that amount until you feel that the fresh or frozen fruit makes it sweet enough. If you're hesitant about the taste of vegetables in a smoothie, start with spinach. Unlike more bitter greens, such as kale and collard greens, spinach has a very subtle flavor, one that is masked easily by the addition of fruit or nut butters. Lastly, all the recipes in this chapter call for nondairy milk to provide more options for those with an allergy or intolerance, but you can certainly use dairy milk if you prefer.

With all this talk about smoothies, you may be wondering about juicing, a trend that is very popular in wellness circles. It's important to know the difference. Vegetable and fruit juices provide water-soluble vitamins such as vitamin C, but where they fall short is the fiber. Fiber provides a wide variety of health benefits, including regulating bowel movements, aiding in weight management, and reducing the risk of hypertension, diabetes, and certain gastrointestinal diseases. The recommended dietary allowance is 38 grams of fiber per day for men and 25 grams per day for women. When you juice fruits and vegetables, you remove all the pulp and skin, which means you lose all that natural dietary fiber. Juicing leaves you with water, sugar, and some (but not all) of a fruit or vegetable's micronutrients. On the other hand, when you blend whole fruits and vegetables in a smoothie, you reap the benefits of consuming all the micronutrients *and* all the natural fiber these foods provide. If you prefer juicing over blending, try using more vegetables such as kale, spinach, celery, parsley, and cucumbers and less fruit such as apples and oranges. This will keep the nutrient content high and sugar content low.

One great thing about smoothies is that they can be made on a budget. The secret? Buy frozen fruit. Not only does this eliminate the need for ice cubes and make for creamier smoothies, but fruit is frozen at peak ripeness, so it contains just as many nutrients as fresh—if not more. Stores like Costco and Trader Joe's, or your local grocery store, should all have a variety of frozen fruit available at affordable prices. You can also buy fresh fruit when it's in season (in other words, at its cheapest) and freeze the fruit yourself in freezer-safe bags or containers. I like to go to my local farmers' market to stock up on fresh blueberries, strawberries, and peaches and keep extras frozen through the winter months.

Some of the add-ins in these recipes may sound expensive, but properly storing spices like ground turmeric or cinnamon can make them last a few years. One bag of Navitas organic ground turmeric is around $8 depending on where you shop, and at 45 servings per bag, this comes out to be just $0.17 per serving. You don't need overpriced superfoods like goji berries, moon juice, and green powders in your smoothies; you get plenty of vitamins and minerals from basic whole foods like vegetables, fruits, nuts, seeds, and spices.

There is one element to smoothie making that I believe is worth the extra cost: a high-speed blender. Vitamix and Blendtec are the top two brands I recommend. While these blenders are more expensive than standard blenders, their durability and powerful blades make them well worth the cost if you plan to make smoothies regularly. They can also double as a food processor, which is a kitchen gadget used in quite a few of the recipes in this cookbook, such as my 3-Ingredient Energy Bars (see page 187), Avocado Mousse (see page 211), Cashew Queso (see page 192), and Basil Pesto (see page 147).

# BUILDING A NUTRITIOUS SMOOTHIE

## 1
### Choose 1½ to 2 cups of a liquid

Coconut water
Dairy milk (1%, 2%, whole)
Freshly squeezed orange or apple juice
Nondairy milk (almond, soy, coconut, cashew)
Water

## 2
### Choose 2 cups of leafy greens

Collard greens
Kale
Romaine lettuce
Spinach
Swiss chard
Watercress

## 3
### Choose 1 to 2 cups of fresh or frozen fruit

Apple          Melon
Avocado        Orange
Banana         Peach
Blueberries    Pear
Kiwi           Pineapple
Mango          Strawberries

## 4
### Choose 1 to 2 tablespoons of nuts or seeds

Almond butter
Chia seeds
Ground flaxseed
Peanut butter
Pistachios
Walnuts

## 5
### Add 1 scoop of protein (optional)

Plant-based protein powder
Whey protein powder

## 6
### Add extra add-ins (1 to 2 teaspoons each)

Cacao powder
Ground cinnamon
Ground ginger
Ground turmeric
Maca powder

Rolled oats (at least ½ cup for weight gain)
Spirulina
Whole-milk Greek yogurt (at least ½ cup for weight gain)

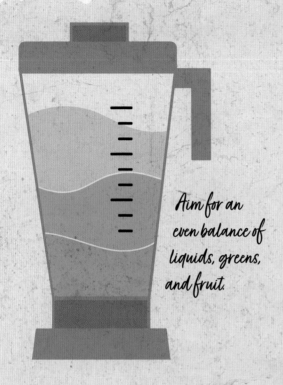

*Aim for an even balance of liquids, greens, and fruit.*

**7**

**Add
6 to 7 ice cubes
(optional)**

**8**

**Blend
until smooth!**

# TROUBLESHOOTING YOUR SMOOTHIE

▶ **If your smoothie is too thick:** Add more liquid and blend for an additional 15 seconds.

▶ **If your smoothie is too thin:** Add more nut butter, fresh fruit, or avocado to thicken it up.

▶ **If your smoothie is too bitter:** Sweeten it with additional fresh or frozen bananas, mango, or pineapple.

▶ **If you need to watch blood sugar levels:** Choose lower-glycemic fruits, such as blueberries, strawberries, raspberries, blackberries, and cherries, and use less than 1 cup. Use an unsweetened nondairy milk, which does not contain sugar, versus dairy milk or juice, which does. Avocados are another good addition to smoothies, as they provide a creamy texture similar to bananas while keeping the sugar content low.

# SIMPLE GREEN SMOOTHIE

DF | GF | NF | V | 30 | NK | OP

MAKES I SERVING

2 cups firmly packed chopped kale

½ green apple, cored and sliced

¼ avocado, pitted and peeled

1 cup unsweetened nondairy milk
or 2% milk

Ice cubes

1 scoop protein powder of choice
(optional)

Put the ingredients in a blender in
the order listed. Blend on high until
smooth.

---

NUTRITION TIP: Only use protein powders that have been verified by a reputable
third-party testing company, such as NSF
Certified for Sport or Informed Sport. Some
examples include Garden of Life Sport, Klean
Athlete, Momentous, Ladder, BiPro, and
NOW Sports.

# BERRY-BEET SMOOTHIE

DF | GF | NF | VEG | 30 | NK | OP

MAKES I SERVING

1 cup unsweetened nondairy milk
or 2% milk

1 cooked beet, chopped

½ cup frozen blueberries

½ cup frozen pineapple chunks

1–2 teaspoons honey

1 scoop protein powder of choice
(optional)

Put the ingredients in a blender in
the order listed. Blend on high until
smooth.

---

COOKING TIP: Cooked beets blend much
more easily than raw. You can find precooked
beets in the produce department at most
grocery stores.

PERFORMANCE TIP: Beet juice has been
shown to help improve stamina and shorten
recovery time between training sessions. This
could be the result of increased blood flow,
allowing for more oxygen to be delivered to
your muscles thanks to the nitrates found
naturally in beets. For the most benefit, drink
30 minutes before your workout.

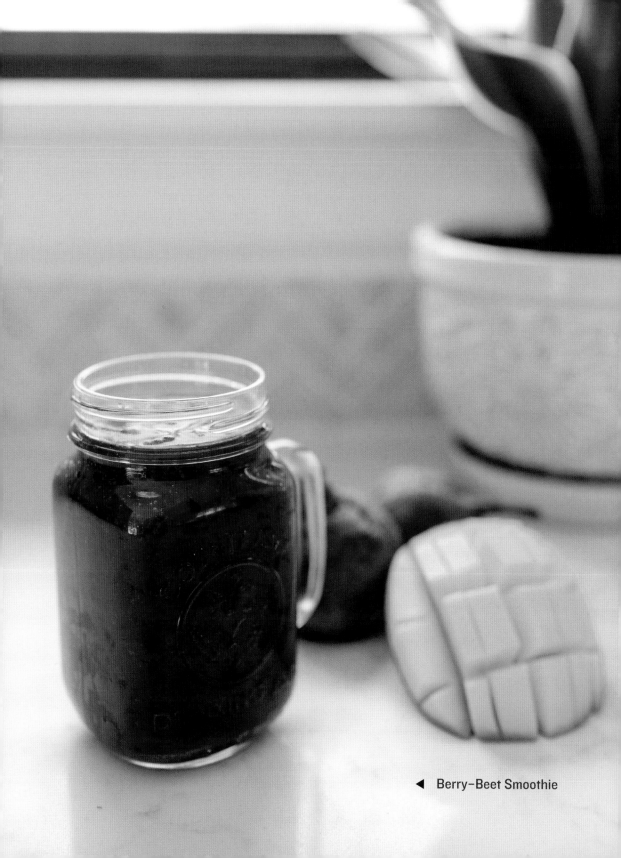

◄ Berry–Beet Smoothie

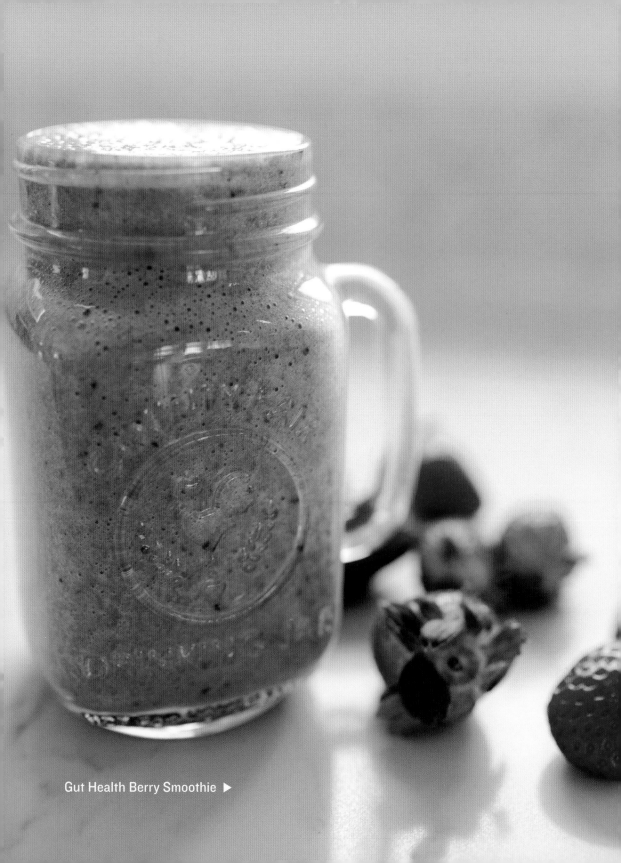

Gut Health Berry Smoothie ▶

# GUT HEALTH BERRY SMOOTHIE

DF | GF | NF | V | 30 | NK | OP

MAKES 1 SERVING

1½ cups unsweetened nondairy milk or 2% milk

1 small frozen banana, chopped

½ cup frozen strawberries, raspberries, or blueberries

¼ cup unsweetened coconut milk yogurt

2 tablespoons ground flaxseed

1 scoop plant-based protein powder of choice

1 cup fresh spinach (optional)

½ teaspoon ground cinnamon (optional)

Put the ingredients in a blender in the order listed. Blend on high until smooth.

---

**PERFORMANCE TIP:** Intense exercise can lead to significant changes within your gut microbiome. Probiotics and prebiotics help keep your gut healthy by promoting the growth of beneficial bacteria. Ground flaxseed and berries provide prebiotics (fiber), and unsweetened coconut milk yogurt is fortified with probiotics (bacteria) to make this smoothie an excellent option to promote optimal gut health.

# TROPICAL GREEN SMOOTHIE

DF | GF | NF | V | 30 | NK | OP

MAKES 1 SERVING

1 cup water or coconut water

2 cups firmly packed fresh spinach

½ cup frozen mango chunks

½ cup frozen pineapple

½ avocado, pitted and peeled, or ½ banana

1 scoop protein powder of choice (optional)

Put the ingredients in a blender in the order listed. Blend on high until smooth.

---

**COOKING TIP:** Using frozen fruit eliminates the need for ice and leaves you with a creamier smoothie.

**PERFORMANCE TIP:** Coconut water is packed with potassium, one of the electrolytes lost in sweat. If you drink this smoothie after a hard workout, add a pinch of salt to up the sodium content.

# CITRUS ANTIOXIDANT SMOOTHIE

DF | GF | NF | V | 30 | NK | OP

MAKES I SERVING

1 cup coconut water or water

2 cups firmly packed fresh spinach

1 orange, peeled

1 cup frozen mango chunks or 1 cup frozen banana slices

1 (1-inch) piece fresh ginger

1 teaspoon ground turmeric

Put the ingredients in a blender in the order listed. Blend on high until smooth.

**NUTRITION TIP:** Citrus fruits are rich in vitamin C, a powerful antioxidant, and turmeric and ginger both offer anti-inflammatory properties. Learn more about antioxidants and anti-inflammatory foods on page 28.

# CHOCOLATE-BANANA SMOOTHIE

DF | GF | V | 30 | NK | OP

MAKES I SERVING

1 cup unsweetened nondairy milk or 2% milk

1 banana

2 tablespoons peanut butter

1 scoop protein powder of choice

1 teaspoon cacao powder

2 cups firmly packed fresh spinach or kale

Ice cubes

Put the ingredients in a blender in the order listed. Blend on high until smooth.

**COOKING TIP:** Cacao powder and cacao nibs are made from fermented, dried, unroasted cacao beans (the same beans used to make chocolate). Cacao powder provides several minerals, including iron, magnesium, and selenium. If you have difficulty finding cacao powder in your grocery store's baking aisle, unsweetened cocoa powder is very similar and would make a great substitute.

**PERFORMANCE TIP:** To increase the calorie and carbohydrate content, add ½ cup old-fashioned rolled oats, an extra banana, and ½ cup additional milk.

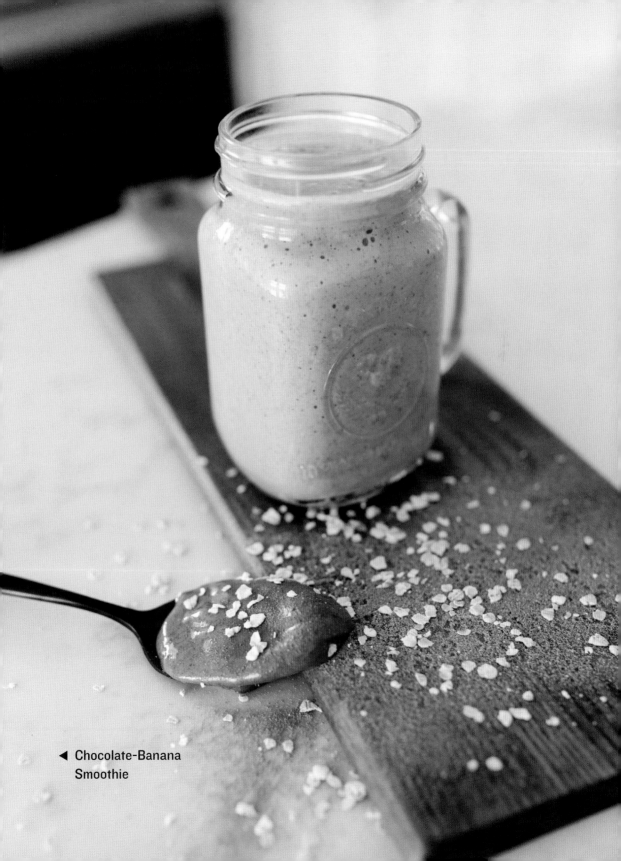

◀ Chocolate-Banana
Smoothie

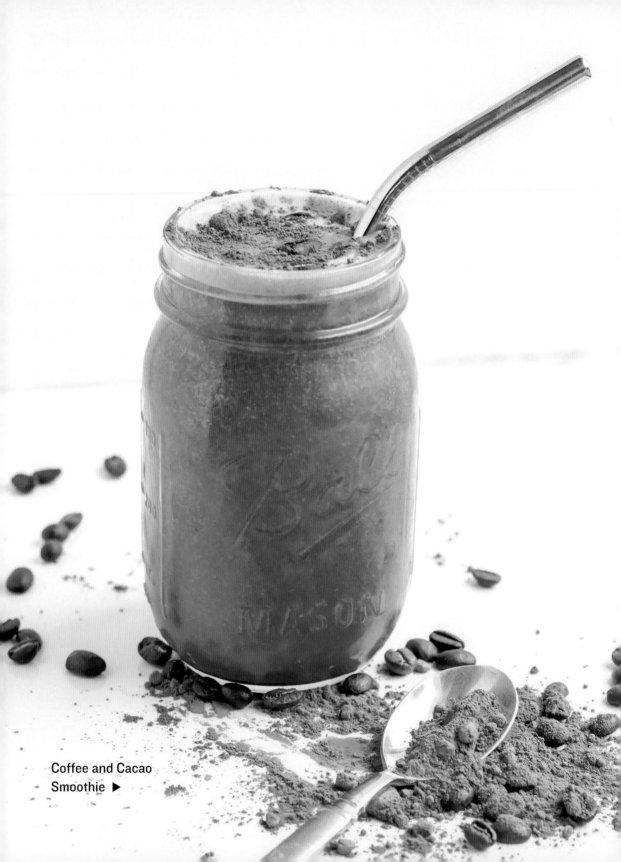

Coffee and Cacao
Smoothie ▶

# PEPPERMINT-CACAO GREEN SMOOTHIE

DF | GF | V | 30 | NK | OP

MAKES 1 SERVING

1 cup unsweetened nondairy milk or 2% milk

1–2 cups firmly packed fresh spinach

1 large frozen banana

1 tablespoon creamy almond butter

2–3 drops (or up to ¼ teaspoon) peppermint extract

¼ teaspoon vanilla extract

3–4 ice cubes

Raw cacao nibs or dark chocolate chips (optional), for topping

Put the ingredients in a blender in the order listed. Blend on high until smooth. Top the smoothie with cacao nibs or chocolate chips (if using).

COOKING TIP: Make sure you use a frozen banana for an extra-creamy consistency.

PERFORMANCE TIP: To boost the protein, add a scoop of vanilla or chocolate protein powder.

# COFFEE AND CACAO SMOOTHIE

DF | GF | V | 30 | NK | OP

MAKES 1 SERVING

1 cup unsweetened vanilla nondairy milk or 2% milk

4–6 ounces cold-brew coffee

1 large frozen banana

1 tablespoon creamy almond butter

3–4 Medjool dates, pitted

1 teaspoon cacao powder

Put the ingredients in a blender in the order listed. Blend on high until smooth.

COOKING TIP: If you prefer a stronger coffee flavor, use more coffee and less milk.

PERFORMANCE TIP: Blood levels of caffeine peak at 45 to 60 minutes post-consumption, so this smoothie would be ideal about an hour before your training session. Choose caffeine from natural sources like coffee or tea that don't contain excess sugar or artificial sweeteners. To boost the protein, add a scoop of chocolate protein powder.

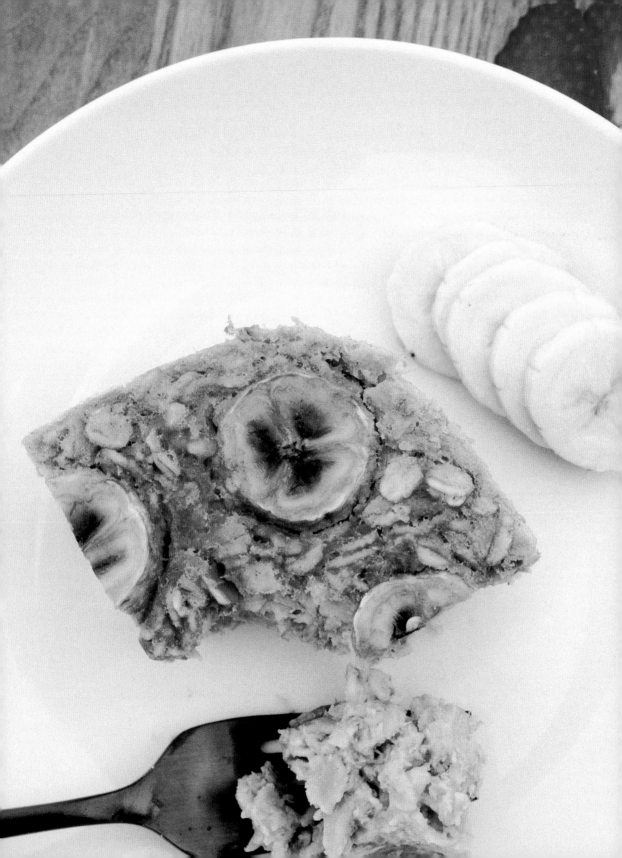

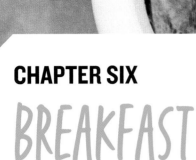

# CHAPTER SIX

# BREAKFAST

For as long as I can remember, breakfast has always been my favorite meal of the day. While I personally lean more toward sweet rather than savory in the mornings, you'll find a variety of both types of dishes in this chapter. If you're someone who doesn't typically eat breakfast, I recommend trying it for three or four days to see how you feel. Chances are, you'll be amazed how much energy and improved concentration you have when you provide your body with a substantial breakfast before a hard training session or long day at work.

A common struggle I hear as to why someone may not eat breakfast is a lack of time in the morning to prepare it. Rest assured that every one of these recipes can be made in advance the night before to take with you on the go the next morning. My favorites for busy mornings are the overnight oats and the baked oatmeal. If you find you don't have much of an appetite in the morning, you might find something lighter, like a small serving of breakfast parfait or chia pudding, to be satisfying. Either way, after you try a few of these recipes, I know you'll have a newfound love for breakfast!

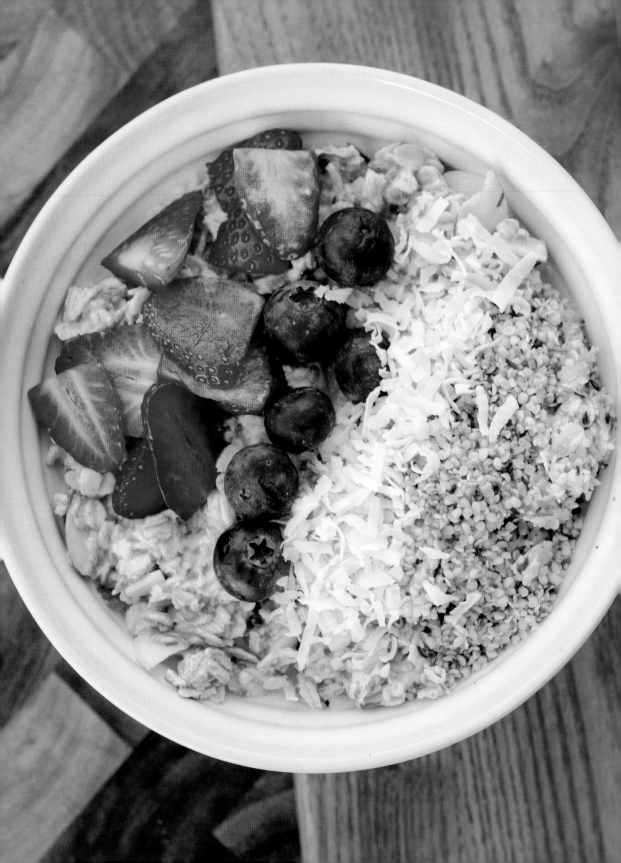

# BASIC OVERNIGHT OATS

DF | GF | V | 30 | NK | OP

½ cup old-fashioned rolled oats

½ cup unsweetened nondairy milk or 2% milk

3 tablespoons sliced almonds or chopped walnuts

1½ teaspoons chia seeds

1 teaspoon pure maple syrup or honey (optional)

1 banana, sliced, or ½ cup blueberries or sliced strawberries

Combine the oats, milk, almonds, chia seeds, and maple syrup (if using) in a glass container. Stir, cover, and store in the refrigerator overnight.

When ready to eat, add the banana and stir again.

---

COOKING TIP: Oats are naturally gluten-free but are often manufactured in facilities that also process gluten-containing grains. For this reason, you will find oats labeled "certified gluten-free," which eliminates the risk of cross-contamination. If you have a food allergy or an intolerance to gluten, make sure to seek out certified gluten-free oats.

# MORNING MUESLI

**DF | VEG | 30 | NK | OP**

MAKES 4 SERVINGS

1 cup old-fashioned rolled oats

1 cup wheat flakes

½ cup chopped pitted dates

½ cup sliced almonds

½ cup sunflower seeds

½ cup raisins

½–1 cup unsweetened nondairy milk or 2% milk

¼ cup finely chopped Granny Smith apple

1 teaspoon honey

Combine the oats, wheat flakes, dates, almonds, sunflower seeds, and raisins in a large container and mix well.

For each serving, measure ½ to 1 cup dry muesli into a bowl and add the milk. Cover and refrigerate overnight. When ready to eat, add the apple and honey.

Store the extra muesli mix in a tightly sealed container at room temperature.

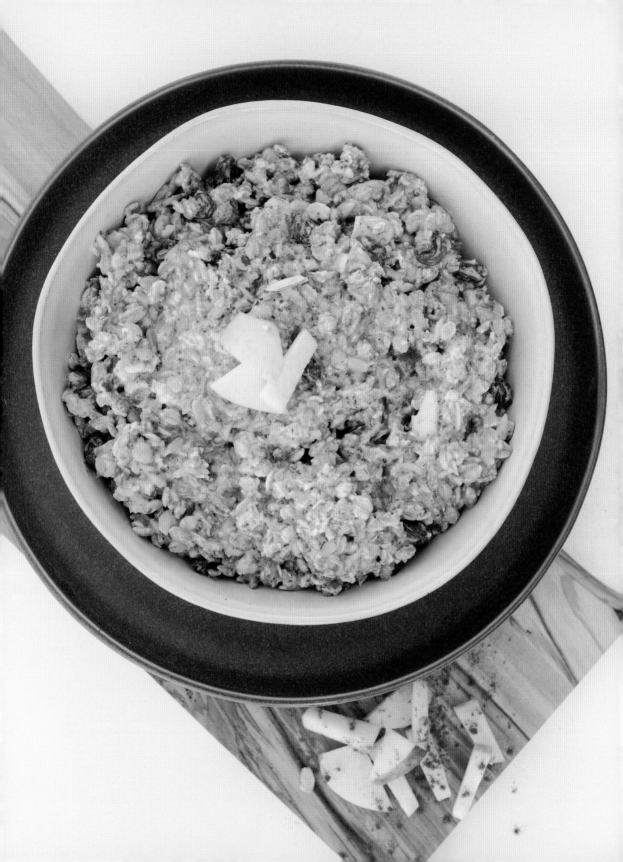

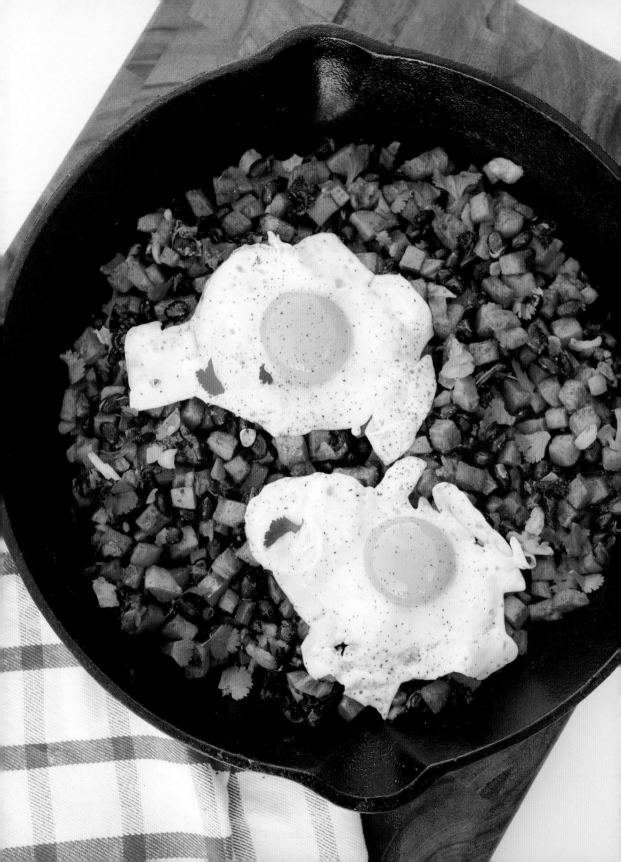

# SWEET POTATO AND BLACK BEAN HASH

**DF | GF | NF | V | 30**

MAKES 4 SERVINGS

2 large sweet potatoes, cut into bite-size pieces

2 tablespoons extra-virgin olive oil, divided

1 teaspoon sweet paprika

1 teaspoon ground cumin

¼ teaspoon ground coriander

¼ teaspoon chili powder

1 cup chopped white onion

1 teaspoon minced garlic

1 (15-ounce) can black beans, drained and rinsed

1 cup firmly packed shredded kale

Salt and black pepper, to taste

Juice of ½ lime

¼ cup chopped fresh cilantro

Preheat the oven to 425°F.

In a large bowl, toss together the sweet potatoes, 1 tablespoon of the oil, the paprika, the cumin, the coriander, and the chili powder. Spread out in a single layer on a rimmed baking sheet and roast for 20 minutes, or until tender.

When the sweet potatoes are nearly done, heat the remaining 1 tablespoon of oil in a large skillet over medium-high heat. Add the onion and sauté for 4 to 5 minutes, until softened. Add the garlic and sauté for 1 minute.

Reduce the heat to medium-low and add the beans and kale. Season with salt and pepper and sauté for a few minutes more, until the kale has wilted.

Add the roasted sweet potatoes to the skillet and stir to combine. Stir in the lime juice and cilantro and serve.

---

**SERVING TIP:** Serve with a fried egg or two on top for additional protein. You can also top with some fresh avocado slices or crumbled goat cheese.

# FARMERS' MARKET EGG CASSEROLE

**GF | NF | VEG**

2 tablespoons avocado oil, divided

3 medium potatoes, shredded, or 3 cups hash browns

½ cup chopped white onion

1 teaspoon minced garlic

½ cup chopped green bell pepper

½ cup chopped white button or cremini mushrooms

9 large eggs

¼ cup unsweetened nondairy milk or 2% milk

¼ cup plus 2 tablespoons shredded cheese of choice

Salt and black pepper, to taste

⅓ cup firmly packed shredded kale

Chopped tomatoes and fresh parsley (optional), for garnish

Preheat the oven to 375°F.

Heat 1 tablespoon of the oil in an 8-inch cast-iron skillet over medium-high heat. Add the potatoes and cook for about 7 minutes, until browned on the bottom. Flip the potatoes and cook for another 2 to 3 minutes, flattening the potatoes on the bottom of the skillet to form a crust.

In a separate skillet, heat the remaining 1 tablespoon of oil over medium-high heat. Add the onion, garlic, bell pepper, and mushrooms and sauté for about 3 minutes, until the onion is translucent. Sprinkle the vegetables evenly on top of the hash browns.

In a mixing bowl, whisk together the eggs, the milk, ¼ cup of the cheese, salt, and pepper. Stir in the kale. Pour the egg mixture on top of the vegetables. Sprinkle the remaining 2 tablespoons of cheese on top.

Bake for 30 to 35 minutes, until the eggs are set. Top with the tomatoes and parsley (if using) and serve.

---

**COOKING TIP:** If you don't have a cast-iron (or other oven-safe) skillet, use a regular skillet and then transfer the ingredients to a casserole dish for baking. Make sure to lightly coat it with more oil (or spray it with olive oil cooking spray) and spread the potatoes out flat on the bottom.

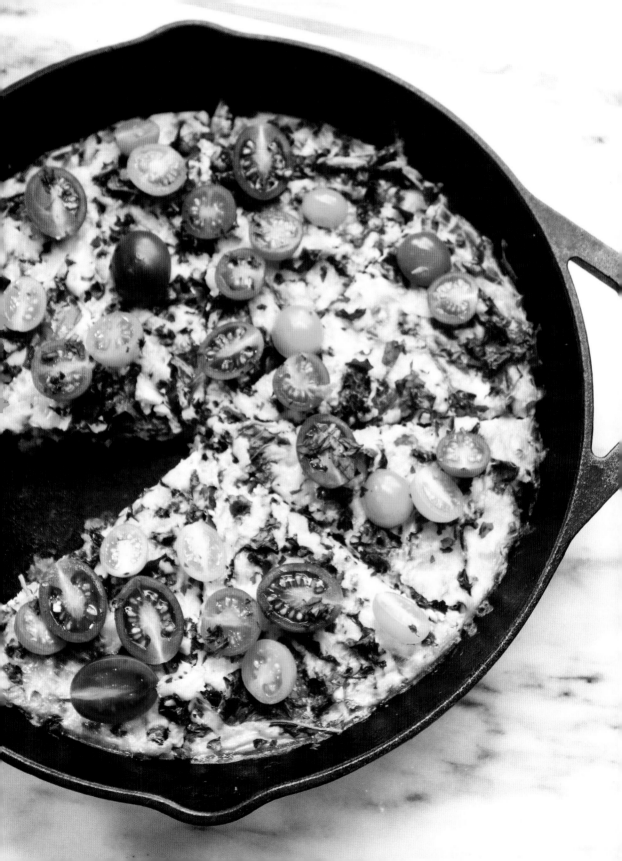

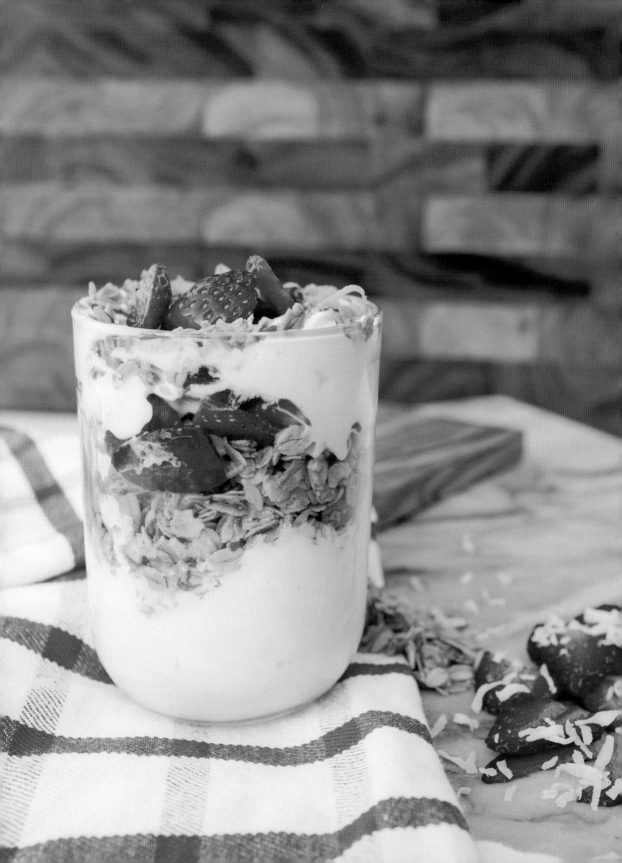

# BREAKFAST PARFAIT

GF | VEG | 30 | NK | OP

1 (5-ounce) container Greek yogurt, skyr, or nondairy yogurt

¼ cup 6-Ingredient Granola (page 97)

¼–1 cup chopped fresh fruit, shredded coconut, and/or nuts

Spoon half of the yogurt into the bottom of a mason jar or bowl. Scatter half of the granola on top, followed by half of the fruit. Repeat the layers.

Serve right away, or cover and store in the refrigerator for up to 5 days.

---

**NUTRITION TIP:** Skip the fat-free flavored yogurt and instead opt for a whole-milk or 2% milk plain Greek yogurt or skyr. Skyr is an Icelandic dairy product with a very similar thick, creamy texture to Greek yogurt. If you find it to be too tart even with the granola and fresh fruit, drizzle a tiny bit of honey on top for added sweetness.

# BAKED OATMEAL CASSEROLE

**DF | GF | VEG | 30**

MAKES 6 SERVINGS

3 cups old-fashioned rolled oats

½ cup chopped walnuts

½ teaspoon ground cinnamon

Pinch of salt

4 ripe bananas

2½ cups unsweetened nondairy milk or 2% milk

1 large egg

⅓ cup creamy peanut butter

2 tablespoons pure maple syrup or honey

Preheat the oven to 350°F. Grease the bottom and sides of a 9 × 9-inch baking pan with olive oil cooking spray.

In a mixing bowl, stir together the oats, walnuts, cinnamon, and salt.

In a separate bowl, use a handheld electric mixer or whisk to combine three of the bananas with the milk, egg, peanut butter, and maple syrup.

Pour the oat mixture into the banana mixture and gently stir together until well combined. Pour the oatmeal mixture into the prepared baking pan and spread it out evenly. Slice the remaining banana and arrange the slices on top of the oatmeal.

Bake for about 30 minutes, until a toothpick inserted into the center of the casserole comes out clean. Serve immediately.

---

**SERVING TIP:** Try serving the casserole with a drizzle of honey, more fresh bananas, or chopped walnuts. To reheat leftovers, microwave for about a minute.

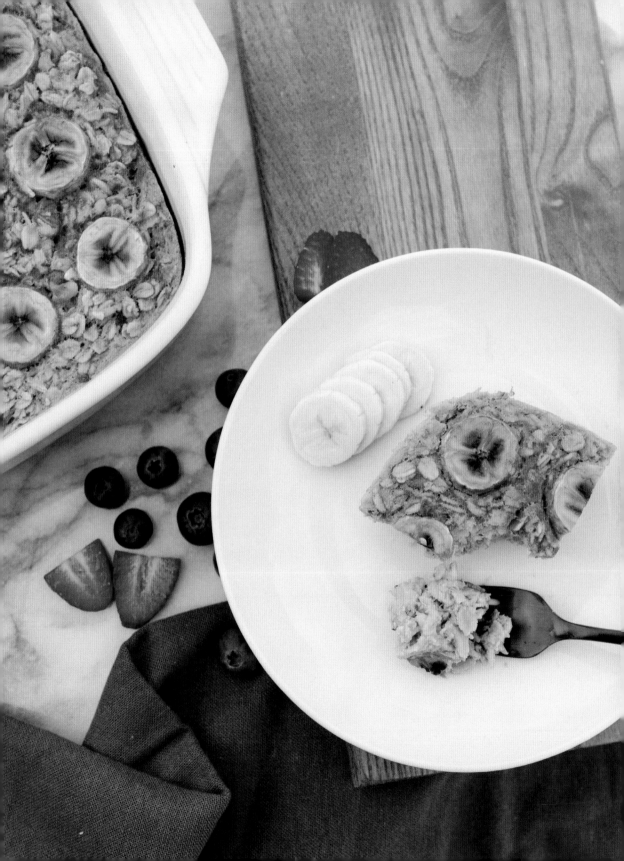

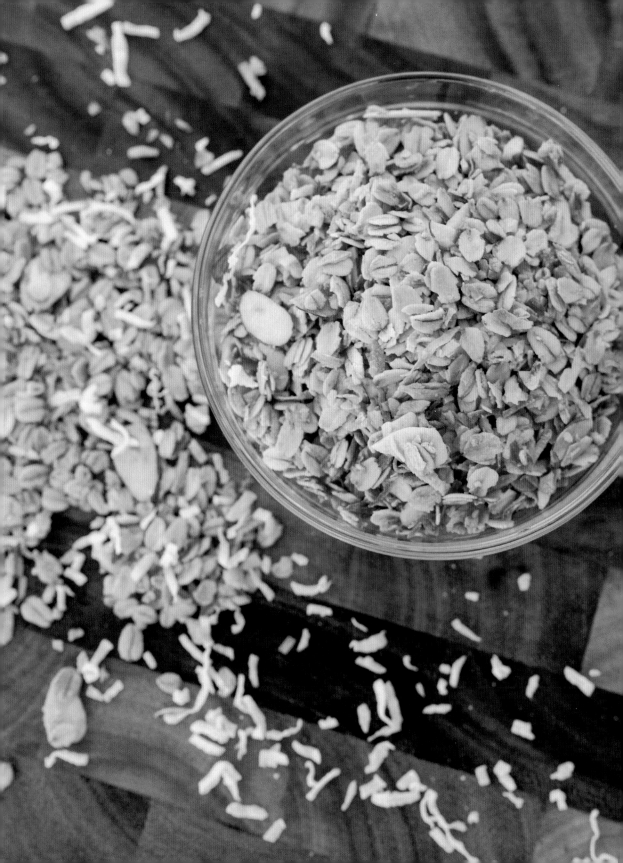

# 6-INGREDIENT GRANOLA

**DF | GF | VEG | 30**

**MAKES 16 (¼-CUP) SERVINGS**

**2 cups old-fashioned rolled oats**

**½ cup unsweetened shredded coconut**

**⅓ cup sliced almonds**

**¼ cup honey**

**2 tablespoons melted coconut oil**

**½ teaspoon vanilla extract**

**3–4 tablespoons finely chopped dried fruit, such as raisins, cherries, apricots, or cranberries (optional)**

Preheat the oven to 325°F.

In a mixing bowl, stir together the oats, coconut, and almonds. Add the honey, oil, and vanilla and mix until well combined.

Spread the mixture into a thin layer on a rimmed baking sheet. Bake for 8 minutes, then stir the granola to prevent burning. Bake for an additional 4 to 6 minutes, until the oats have turned golden brown, checking and stirring every minute to prevent burning.

Let the granola cool, then transfer to an airtight container and store at room temperature for up to 2 weeks. Serve with the dried fruit (if using).

---

**COOKING TIP:** Coconut oil is solid at room temperature and has a melting point around 76°F. Before adding the oil to this recipe, it will need to be melted to allow for easier mixing. You can do this by putting the coconut oil in a small bowl and microwaving for 10-second intervals until it has completely melted.

# CHIA PUDDING

**DF | GF | NF | V | NK | OP**

¼ cup chia seeds

1½ cups unsweetened vanilla nondairy milk or 2% milk

1 tablespoon unsweetened plain coconut milk yogurt (optional)

2 teaspoons pure maple syrup or honey

Combine the chia seeds, milk, yogurt (if using), and maple syrup in an airtight container. Cover and give it a good shake, then refrigerate for about 1 hour. Give it another good shake, then refrigerate for at least 3 more hours, until the chia seeds soak up the milk and the mixture has a consistency similar to tapioca pudding.

To serve, top each serving with one of the fruit and nut variations below. Store leftovers in the refrigerator for up to 5 days.

### TROPICAL CHIA PUDDING VARIATION:

Top the pudding base with ½ cup finely chopped fresh mango or pineapple and 2 tablespoons macadamia nuts.

### KIWI-BERRY CHIA PUDDING VARIATION:

Top the pudding base with ¼ cup fresh blueberries, ¼ cup finely chopped kiwi, and 2 tablespoons sliced almonds.

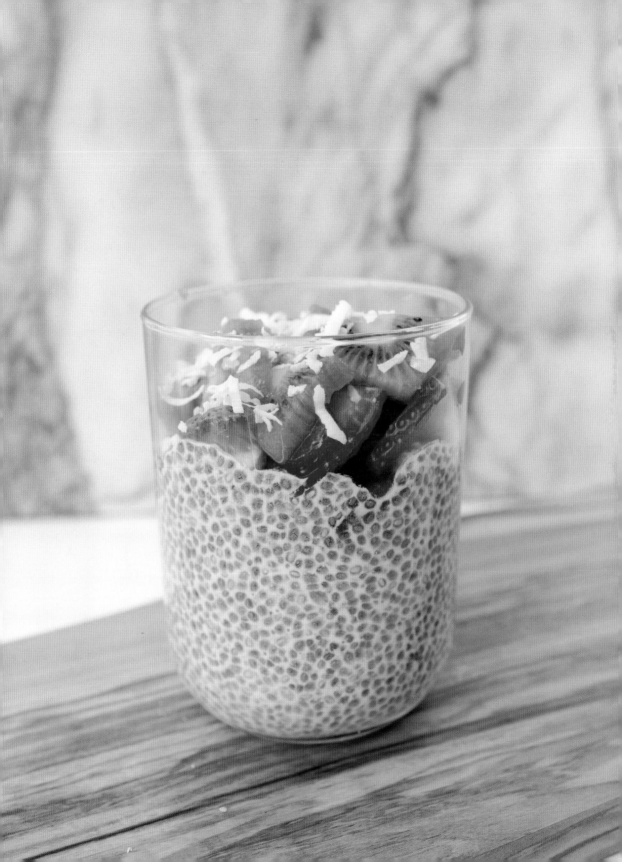

# PRESSURE COOKER FRITTATA

DF | GF | NF | VEG | 30 | NK

9 large eggs

½ cup loosely packed chopped fresh spinach

¼ cup chopped tomato

¼ cup chopped green bell pepper

¼ cup chopped white onion

3 tablespoons shredded cheddar cheese (optional)

½ teaspoon garlic powder

½ teaspoon salt

½ teaspoon black pepper

Place a trivet in an electric pressure cooker and pour in about 1 cup of water. Coat the bottom and sides of a stackable electric pressure cooker pan lightly with olive oil cooking spray.

In a large mixing bowl, beat the eggs. Add the spinach, tomato, bell pepper, onion, cheese (if using), garlic powder, salt, and pepper. Pour the egg mixture into the prepared pan and cover with aluminum foil.

Carefully place the pan on top of the trivet in the pressure cooker. Lock the lid in place and turn the valve to the sealing position. Select the "manual/pressure cook" function and set to 5 minutes. When the cooking time is up, let the pressure cooker naturally release pressure for 10 minutes, then flip the valve to the venting position. Remove the frittata and serve.

COOKING TIP: This frittata can also be made in a slow cooker. Lightly grease the slow cooker with olive oil cooking spray. Add the egg mixture, cover, and cook on low for 2½ hours.

# NO-SUGAR-ADDED ACAI BOWL

**DF | GF | V | 30 | NK | OP**

1 (3.5-ounce) packet frozen unsweetened acai berry puree

½ frozen banana

¼ cup frozen mango chunks

½ cup unsweetened vanilla nondairy milk or 2% milk

½ fresh banana, sliced

¼ cup blueberries

¼ cup chopped walnuts

1 tablespoon unsweetened coconut flakes

1 teaspoon almond butter

1 teaspoon chia seeds

Combine the acai berry, frozen banana, mango, and milk in a blender. Blend on high until smooth, then transfer to a serving bowl. Top with the fresh banana, blueberries, walnuts, coconut, almond butter, and chia seeds and serve.

---

**NUTRITION TIP:** Acai berries contain antioxidants, but traditional acai bowls sold at smoothie and juice bars are typically very high in added sugar. Here we use naturally sweet fruit to add sweetness.

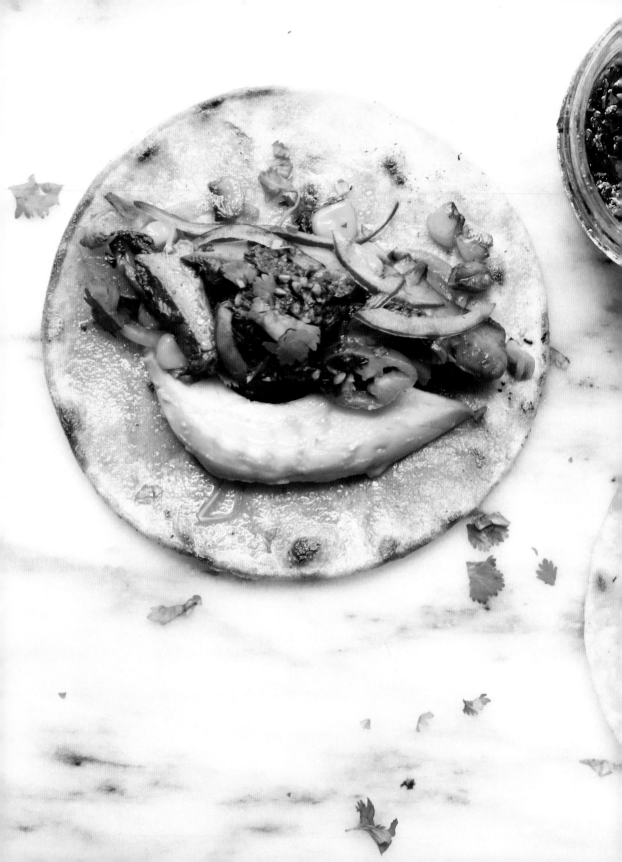

# CHAPTER SEVEN

# SALADS, SOUPS, BOWLS, AND HANDHELDS

Some of my all-time favorite dishes are in this chapter. It's very rare that an entire week goes by that I don't have an anti-inflammatory salad or Buddha bowl for lunch and either lentil tacos or chickpea-lentil curry for dinner. These are my staples, and I believe they may quickly become yours, too. The buffalo chicken tacos and chicken burrito bowls are two favorites among my clients. Whether you're a vegan, a vegetarian, or a meat eater, there's a recipe here just for you.

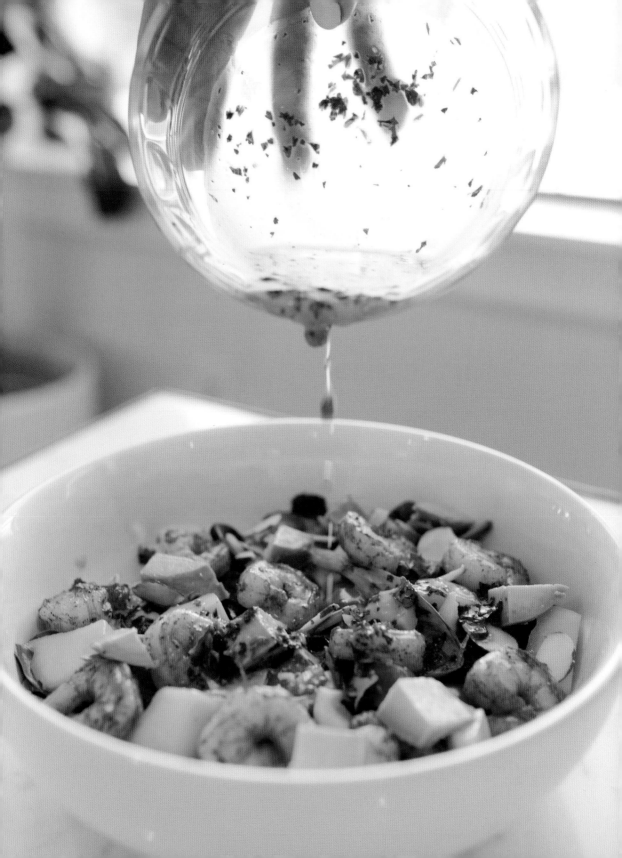

# GRILLED SHRIMP AND MANGO SALAD WITH CILANTRO-LIME VINAIGRETTE

DF | GF | 30

MAKES 2 SERVINGS

1 tablespoon extra-virgin olive oil

8 ounces raw shrimp, peeled and deveined

¼ teaspoon ground cumin

¼ teaspoon chili powder

Salt and black pepper, to taste

4 cups firmly packed spring mix or romaine lettuce

1 mango, pitted, peeled, and chopped

½ avocado, pitted, peeled, and sliced

½ cup sliced cherry tomatoes

2 tablespoons sliced almonds

Cilantro-Lime Vinaigrette (recipe follows), for serving

Heat the oil in a large skillet over medium-high heat. Add the shrimp, then sprinkle on the cumin, chili powder, salt, and pepper. Cook the shrimp on each side for about 3 minutes, until no longer pink.

In a large serving bowl, toss together the spring mix, mango, avocado, and tomatoes. Add the shrimp and almonds. Drizzle with the vinaigrette and serve.

## CILANTRO-LIME VINAIGRETTE

DF | GF | NF | VEG | 30 | NK | OP

MAKES ¼ CUP

Juice of 1 lime

2 tablespoons extra-virgin olive oil

1 tablespoon honey

¼ cup chopped fresh cilantro

Pinch of salt

Put all the ingredients in a blender or food processor. Blend until well combined. Store in an airtight container in the refrigerator for up to 2 weeks.

# ANTI-INFLAMMATORY SALAD WITH HONEY-LEMON VINAIGRETTE

DF | GF | VEG | 30 | NK | OP

**MAKES 4 SERVINGS**

6 cups chopped kale

1 cucumber, chopped

2 stalks celery, chopped

1 cup fresh blueberries

1 apple, cored and sliced

1 avocado, pitted, peeled, and sliced

½ cup chopped walnuts

Honey-Lemon Vinaigrette (recipe follows), for serving

In a large serving bowl, toss together the kale, cucumber, celery, blueberries, apple, avocado, and walnuts. Drizzle with the vinaigrette and serve.

---

**PERFORMANCE TIP:** To boost the carbohydrate content of this salad, add ½ cup cold cooked quinoa. I like to make a large batch of quinoa or rice on the weekend and keep it in my fridge to sprinkle on top of salads throughout the week. For additional protein, top the salad with Roasted Chickpeas (see page 191), two hard-boiled eggs, a handful of edamame, or a slice of leftover Simple Baked Salmon (see page 144).

## HONEY-LEMON VINAIGRETTE

DF | GF | NF | VEG | 30 | NK | OP

**MAKES ¼ CUP**

3 tablespoons extra-virgin olive oil

2 teaspoons honey

2 teaspoons apple cider vinegar

Juice of ½ lemon

Salt and black pepper, to taste

In a small bowl, whisk together all the ingredients. Store in an airtight container in the refrigerator for up to 2 weeks.

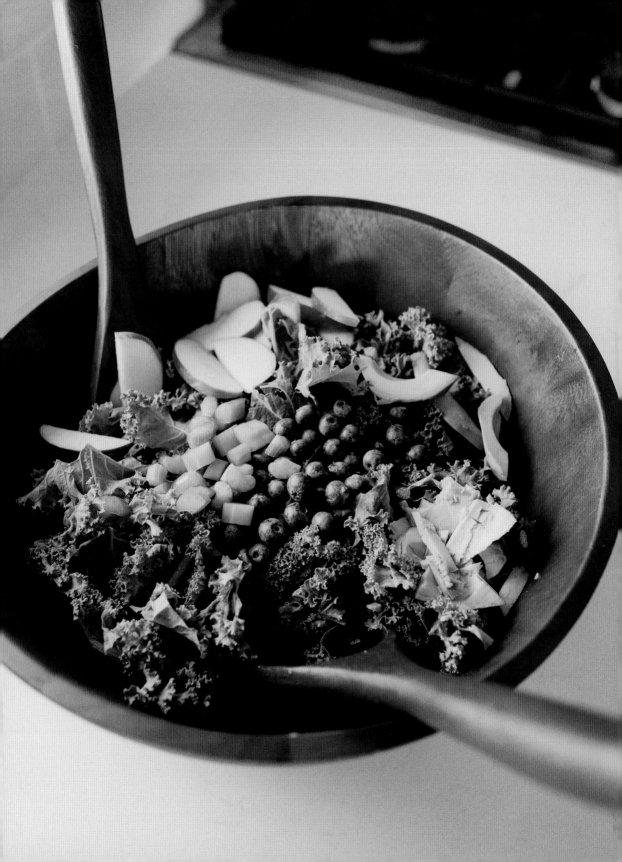

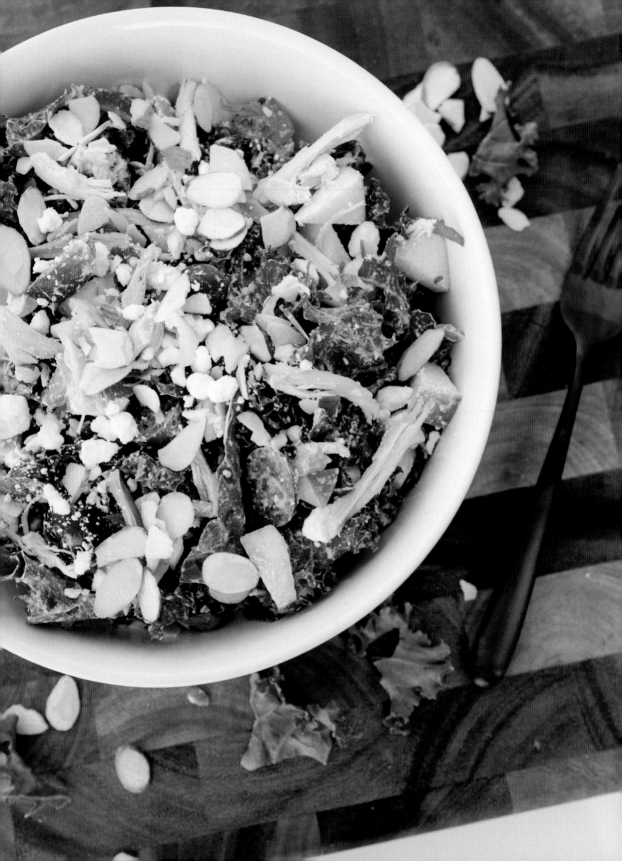

# WALDORF KALE SALAD WITH YOGURT DRESSING

GF | VEG | 30 | NK | OP

MAKES 2 SERVINGS

2 cups firmly packed shredded kale

1 apple, cored and chopped

½ cup grapes, halved

½ cup chopped celery

¼ cup crumbled goat cheese or gorgonzola

¼ cup sliced almonds or chopped walnuts

Yogurt Dressing (recipe follows), for serving

In a large bowl, toss together the kale, apple, grapes, celery, cheese, and almonds. Drizzle with the dressing and serve.

---

**PERFORMANCE TIP:** To boost the protein of this salad, add cooked chicken, edamame, hard-boiled egg, or chickpeas. The salad shown here is topped with rotisserie chicken.

---

## YOGURT DRESSING

GF | NF | VEG | 30 | NK | OP

MAKES ¼ CUP

3 tablespoons plain Greek yogurt

2 teaspoons honey

1 teaspoon mustard

Sea salt and black pepper, to taste

Water, as needed

In a small bowl, whisk together the yogurt, honey, mustard, salt, and pepper. Add water, a teaspoon at a time, until the dressing is pourable but still creamy. Store in an airtight container in the refrigerator for up to 1 week.

# SOUTHWEST CHICKEN SOUP

**DF | GF | NF | NK | OP**

MAKES 5 SERVINGS

1 pound boneless, skinless chicken breasts

1 (28-ounce) can diced tomatoes, undrained

1 (15-ounce) can black beans, rinsed and drained

1 (4-ounce) can chopped green chiles, drained

1 cup frozen corn

1 medium white onion, chopped

1 green bell pepper, seeded and chopped

1 jalapeño, seeded if desired and minced

1 teaspoon minced garlic

3 cups low-sodium chicken broth

1½ teaspoons ground cumin

1½ teaspoons chili powder

¼ teaspoon sea salt

¼ teaspoon black pepper

Sliced avocado, shredded cheese, and/or tortilla strips, for topping (optional)

Put the chicken breasts in a slow cooker. Add the diced tomatoes with their juices, beans, chiles, corn, onion, bell pepper, jalapeño, garlic, broth, cumin, chili powder, salt, and pepper. Cover and cook on high for 3 to 4 hours or on low for 6 to 7 hours, until the chicken is cooked through.

Transfer the chicken to a cutting board. Use two forks to shred the chicken, then return the shredded chicken to the slow cooker, stirring to mix well.

Ladle into bowls and serve with avocado, cheese, and tortilla strips (if using).

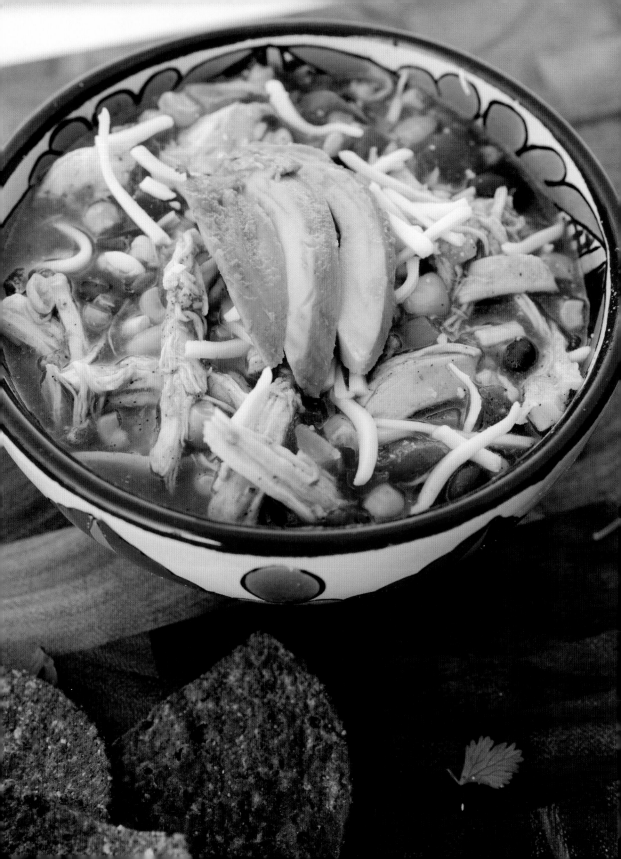

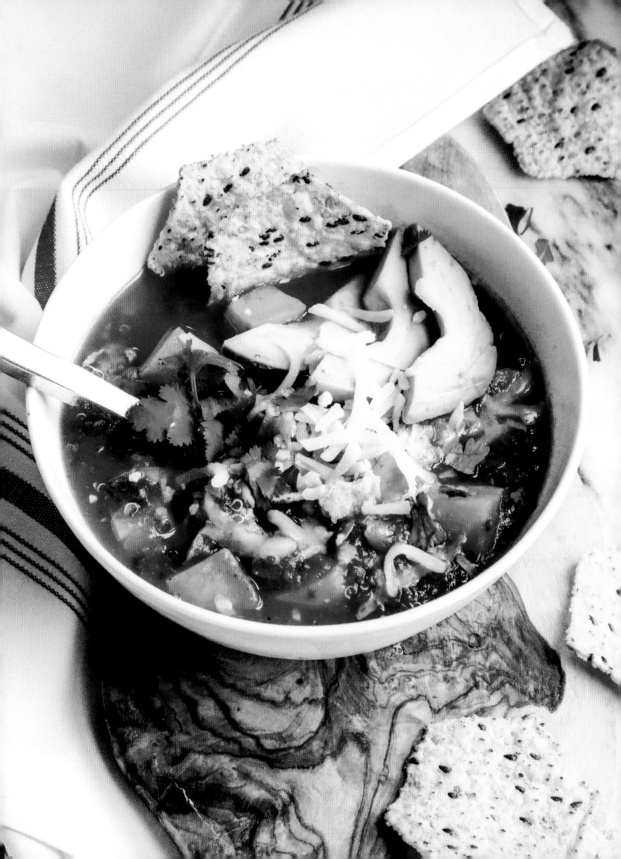

# SWEET POTATO AND TURKEY CHILI

**DF | GF | NF**

1 tablespoon extra-virgin olive oil

1 pound lean ground turkey

1 large sweet potato, peeled and chopped

1 medium white onion, chopped

1 green bell pepper, seeded and chopped

1–2 tablespoons minced garlic

3 cups low-sodium chicken or vegetable broth

1 (28-ounce) can crushed tomatoes

1 (16-ounce) can black beans, rinsed and drained

½ cup uncooked quinoa, rinsed

2 tablespoons chili powder

1 teaspoon ground cumin

½ teaspoon smoked paprika

¼ teaspoon salt

¼ teaspoon black pepper

¼ teaspoon cayenne pepper

Sliced avocado, shredded cheese, and/or whole-grain crackers, for serving (optional)

Heat the oil in a large skillet over medium-high heat. Add the turkey and cook, breaking the meat up with a spoon, for 5 minutes, or until no longer pink.

Transfer the turkey to a slow cooker. Add the sweet potato, onion, bell pepper, garlic, broth, tomatoes, beans, quinoa, chili powder, cumin, paprika, salt, black pepper, and cayenne, stirring to mix well.

Cover and cook on high for 3 to 4 hours or on low for 6 to 8 hours, stirring once or twice, until the sweet potatoes are tender.

Ladle into bowls and serve with avocado, cheese, and crackers (if using).

---

**NUTRITION TIP:** Sweet potatoes are rich in beta-carotene, and quinoa provides magnesium, iron, fiber, and zinc. Both are added to this chili not just for the nutrients but for the texture and flavor they provide. The quinoa especially makes for a delicious, heartier chili.

# LENTIL CHILI

**DF | GF | NF | V | NK | OP**

MAKES 6 SERVINGS

½ cup uncooked quinoa, rinsed

½ cup uncooked green lentils

1 (15-ounce) can black beans, rinsed and drained

1 (15-ounce) can diced tomatoes, undrained

1 (15-ounce) can tomato sauce

4 cups low-sodium vegetable broth

1 small white onion, chopped

1 green bell pepper, seeded and chopped

1 jalapeño, seeded if desired and minced, or 1 teaspoon red pepper flakes (optional)

2 teaspoons minced garlic

1½ tablespoons chili powder

1½ teaspoons ground cumin

1 teaspoon dried oregano

¾ teaspoon sea salt

1 teaspoon black pepper

¼ teaspoon cayenne pepper

Sliced avocado, for serving

Combine the quinoa, lentils, beans, diced tomatoes with their juices, tomato sauce, broth, onion, bell pepper, jalapeño (if using), garlic, chili powder, cumin, oregano, salt, black pepper, and cayenne in a slow cooker, stirring to combine.

Cover and cook on low for 5 to 6 hours, until the lentils are tender.

Ladle into bowls and serve with avocado.

# CHICKPEA-LENTIL CURRY

DF | GF | NF | V

MAKES 4 SERVINGS

2 tablespoons extra-virgin olive oil

1½ teaspoons minced garlic

2 large carrots, chopped

2 (15-ounce) cans chickpeas, rinsed and drained

2 teaspoons ground turmeric

2 teaspoons tikka seasoning, such as Spicemode

½ teaspoon sea salt

½ teaspoon black pepper

½ teaspoon red pepper flakes, or to taste

3 cups vegetable broth

1⅔ cups canned full-fat coconut milk

½ cup uncooked green lentils

1 cup uncooked basmati rice

1¾ cups water

1 cup packed chopped kale

Heat the oil in a large pot over medium-high heat. Add the garlic and carrots and sauté for about 3 minutes. Add the chickpeas, turmeric, tikka seasoning, salt, black pepper, and red pepper flakes, stirring well. Cook for 6 to 7 minutes, until the chickpeas are slightly browned and crispy.

Add the broth, coconut milk, and lentils. Reduce the heat to medium-low and simmer, stirring occasionally, for 20 minutes.

While the curry is simmering, combine the rice and water in a medium saucepan. Bring to a boil over high heat. Reduce the heat to a low simmer, cover, and cook for about 20 minutes, or until the water is absorbed and the rice is tender. (After cooking, you can stir in 1 tablespoon additional coconut milk for a creamier texture and flavor.)

When the curry is done, stir in the kale and cook for about 4 minutes, until the kale is wilted.

Serve the curry on top of the rice.

---

PERFORMANCE TIP: This dish already provides 21 grams of protein per serving, but if you are not vegan/vegetarian, you could throw in some shrimp for even more protein.

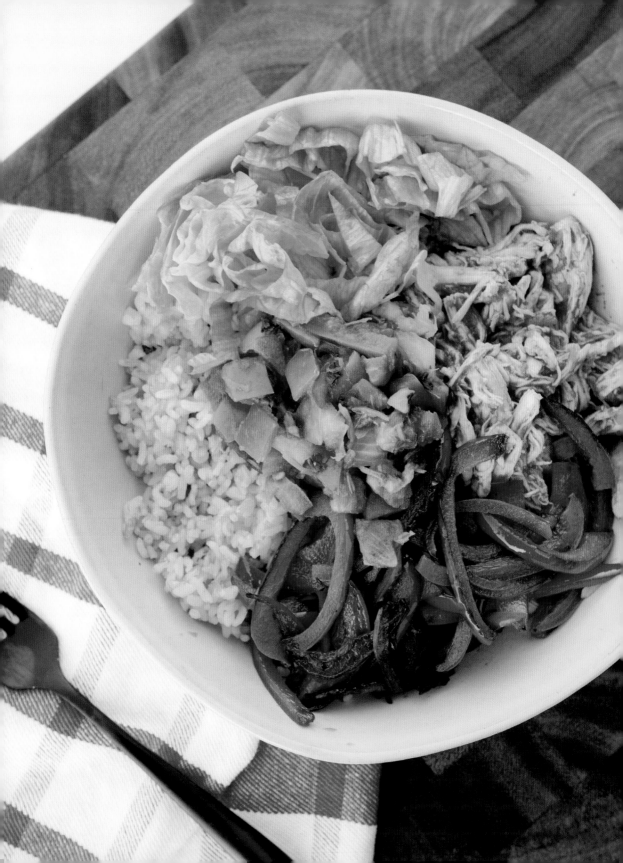

# SHREDDED SALSA CHICKEN BURRITO BOWLS

**DF | GF | NF | NK**

MAKES 8 SERVINGS

2 pounds boneless, skinless chicken breasts

1 (15-ounce) jar salsa

4 cups cooked brown rice

1 (15-ounce) can black beans, rinsed and drained

1 (10-ounce) bag shredded romaine lettuce

1 large tomato, chopped

1 red or green bell pepper, sliced

Guacamole or sliced avocado, for serving (optional)

If using a **slow cooker**, put the chicken breasts in the slow cooker and cover them with the salsa. Cover and cook on high for 3 hours or on low for 5 to 6 hours, until the chicken is cooked through.

If using an **electric pressure cooker**, put the chicken breasts in the pressure cooker and cover them with the salsa. Lock the lid in place and turn the valve to the sealing position. Select the "manual/pressure cook" function and set to 14 minutes. When the cooking time is up, let the pressure cooker naturally release pressure for 10 minutes, then flip the valve to the venting position.

Transfer the chicken to a cutting board. Use two forks to shred the chicken. Return the chicken to the pot, stir to combine, and let sit for 5 minutes.

Portion the rice and beans into bowls. Add the chicken and top with the romaine, tomato, and bell pepper. Serve with guacamole (if using).

---

**COOKING TIP:** Purchase frozen cooked rice and reheat it in a microwave. If you have access to a stove, try sautéing the bell pepper in a bit of olive oil for more flavor before serving.

# RAMEN BOWLS

**DF | GF | NF | VEG | 30**

MAKES 2 SERVINGS

1 (15-ounce) package extra-firm tofu

2 large eggs

1 tablespoon toasted sesame oil or extra-virgin olive oil

1 cup sliced shiitake mushrooms

2 tablespoons tamari or coconut aminos

1 (2.8-ounce) package Lotus Foods Millet & Brown Rice Ramen with Miso Soup

2 cups low-sodium vegetable or mushroom broth

Chopped scallions and sesame seeds, for topping (optional)

To press the tofu, wrap it in a clean dish towel or paper towels and place something heavy (such as a cast-iron skillet) on top. Let it drain for 15 minutes. (Pressing helps remove moisture from the tofu, allowing it to soak up more flavor.)

Meanwhile, put the eggs in a small saucepan and cover with water. Bring to a boil over high heat. Boil the eggs for 4 minutes, then immediately transfer them to a bowl of ice-cold water to cool. Peel the eggs and slice in half lengthwise.

Unwrap the tofu and cut it into bite-size pieces.

Heat the oil in a skillet over medium-high heat. Add the tofu and mushrooms and sauté until lightly browned, about 6 minutes. Reduce the heat to low and add the tamari.

Cook the noodles according to the package directions and drain. Return the noodles to the pot and add the broth and the flavor packet. Bring to a simmer for about 4 minutes.

Divide the noodles and broth between two bowls. Top with the tofu, mushrooms, and eggs. Sprinkle with the scallions and sesame seeds (if using) and serve.

---

**COOKING TIP:** Tamari is a gluten-free alternative to soy sauce. While it's still made from soy, it does not contain any wheat. If you don't like tofu, you can use chopped boneless, skinless chicken breast or shrimp instead.

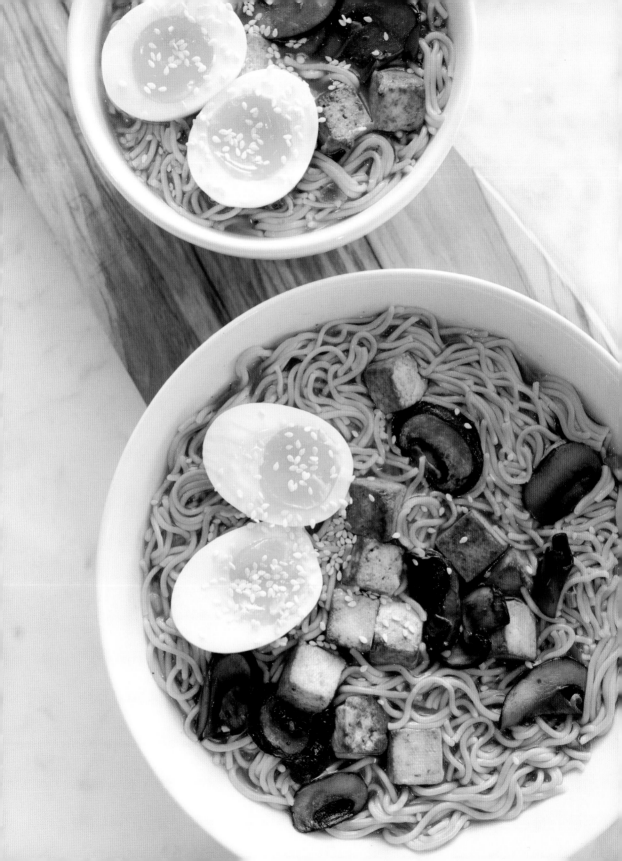

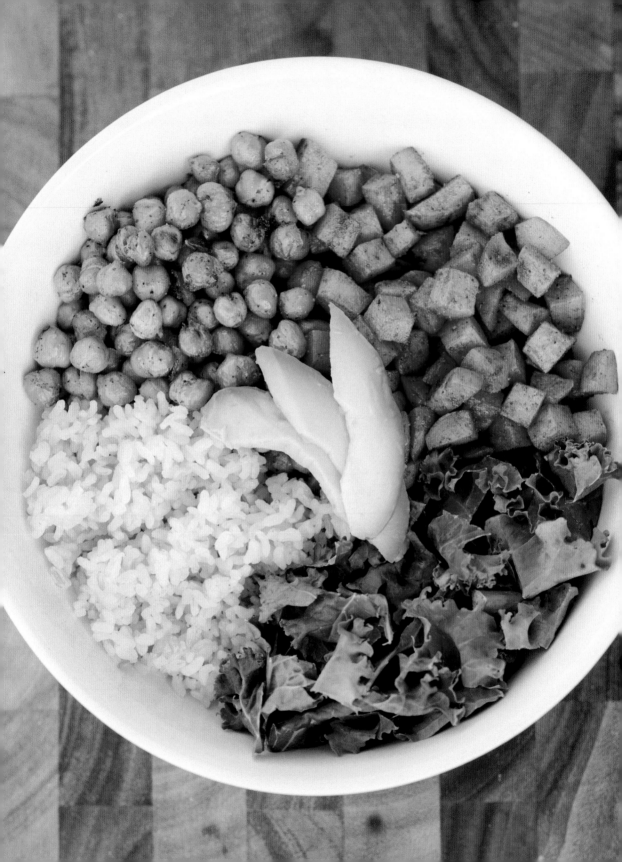

# VEGAN BUDDHA BOWLS

**DF | GF | NF | V**

**MAKES 2-3 SERVINGS**

### Sweet Potatoes

**2 medium sweet potatoes, peeled and chopped**

**2 tablespoons extra-virgin olive oil or avocado oil**

**2 teaspoons chili powder**

**1 teaspoon sweet paprika**

**½ teaspoon garlic powder**

**½ teaspoon ground cumin**

**¼ teaspoon sea salt**

### Chickpeas

**1 (15-ounce) can chickpeas, rinsed, drained, and patted dry**

**2 teaspoons extra-virgin olive oil or avocado oil**

**½ teaspoon chili powder**

**¼ teaspoon sea salt**

### For serving

**1 cup cooked whole grains, such as rice, quinoa, or buckwheat**

**2 cups chopped raw leafy greens, such as kale, spinach, or arugula**

**1 small avocado, pitted, peeled, and sliced**

**Dressing of choice**

Preheat the oven to 400°F. Line two baking sheets with parchment paper or aluminum foil.

In a large mixing bowl, toss the sweet potatoes with the oil, chili powder, paprika, garlic powder, cumin, and salt. Spread out the seasoned potatoes in a single layer on one prepared baking sheet. Roast for 15 minutes, flip the potatoes, then roast for another 15 to 20 minutes, until the potatoes are lightly browned.

At the same time, spread out the chickpeas on the other prepared baking sheet. Roast for about 35 minutes, shaking the pan every 10 minutes, until the chickpeas are lightly browned. Transfer to a large bowl and add the oil, chili powder, and salt.

Divide the sweet potatoes, chickpeas, grains, and greens between two bowls. Add the avocado on top and drizzle with dressing. Serve.

---

**COOKING TIP:** I prefer to season the chickpeas after roasting for a more intense flavor, but you can definitely do this step prior to roasting if you prefer.

# BUFFALO CHICKEN TACOS WITH RANCH DRESSING

GF | NF | 30

6 small corn or flour tortillas

½ recipe Shredded Buffalo Chicken (page 159)

2 stalks celery, finely chopped

2 large carrots, finely chopped

Buffalo sauce, such as The New Primal, for serving

Ranch Dressing (recipe follows) or store-bought ranch dressing, for serving

Warm up each tortilla in a skillet over low heat for about 30 seconds on each side.

To assemble the tacos, fill each tortilla with some chicken, celery, and carrots. Drizzle buffalo sauce and ranch on top. Serve.

---

COOKING TIP: To make this recipe dairy-free, omit the ranch dressing or purchase a dairy-free ranch dressing, such as Tessemae's.

## RANCH DRESSING

MAKES ¾ CUP

GF | NF | VEG | 30 | NK | OP

½ cup plain Greek yogurt

1 teaspoon dried dill

2 tablespoons extra-virgin olive oil

2 tablespoons grated parmesan cheese

1 clove garlic

Pinch of sea salt and black pepper

Combine all the ingredients in a food processor and blend until smooth. Refrigerate in an airtight container for up to 1 week.

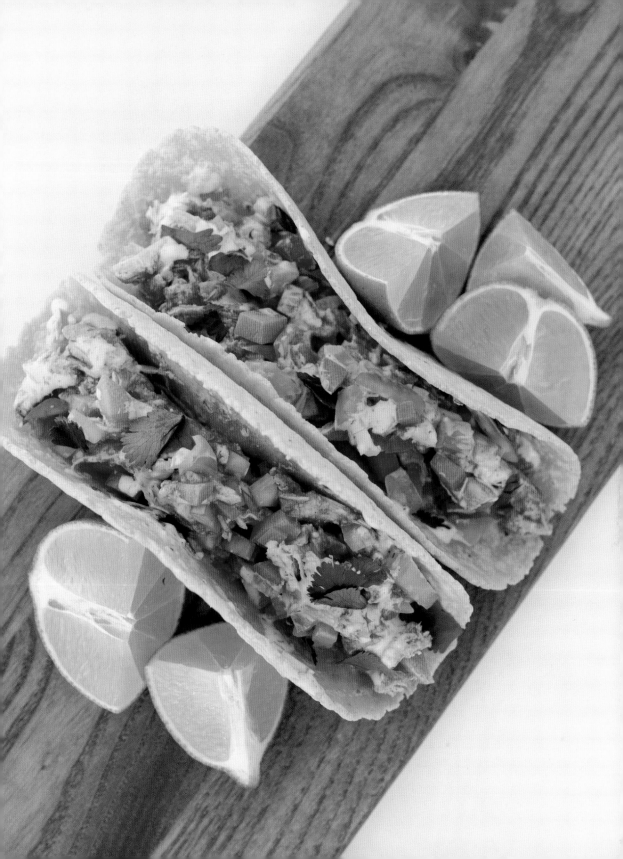

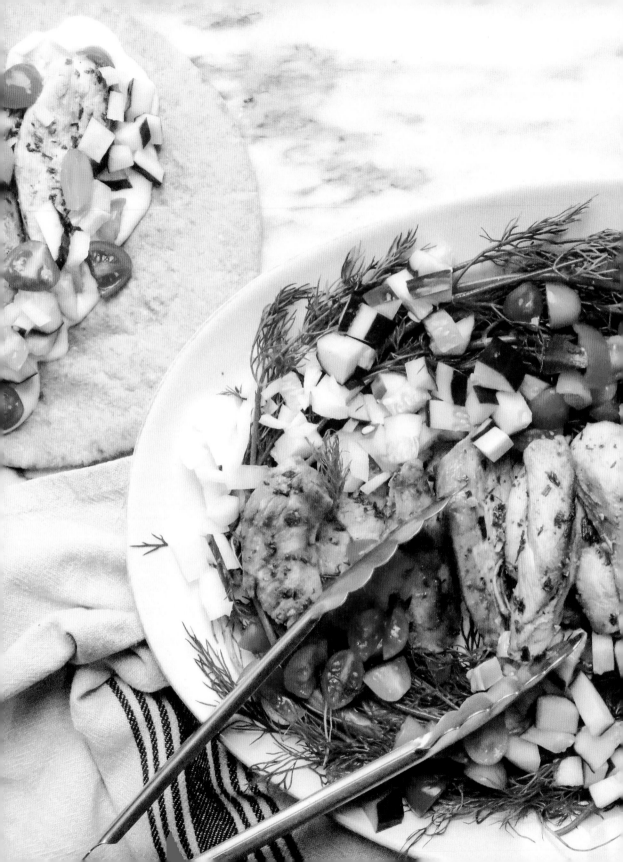

# CHICKEN GYROS

**NF | 30**

MAKES 4 SERVINGS

4 whole-wheat pitas

⅔ recipe Mediterranean Chicken (page 163)

½ large cucumber, chopped

1 cup grape tomatoes, chopped

½ medium white onion, chopped

Tzatziki Sauce (recipe follows), for serving

Feta cheese, for serving (optional)

Warm up each pita in a skillet over low heat for 2 to 3 minutes.

Fill each pita with some of the chicken. Top with the cucumber, tomatoes, onion, and 1 to 2 tablespoons of the tzatziki sauce. Add a spoonful of feta cheese (if using) and serve.

---

**COOKING TIP:** Be sure to peel and seed the cucumber before blending, as leaving the seeds in can result in a watery tzatziki sauce.

## TZATZIKI SAUCE

**GF | NF | VEG | 30**

MAKES 1½ CUPS

1 cup plain Greek yogurt

1 large cucumber, peeled and seeded

1½ teaspoons dried dill or 1 tablespoon fresh dill

1 clove garlic

½ teaspoon black pepper

Pinch of sea salt

Combine all the ingredients in a food processor and blend until smooth. Store in an airtight container in the refrigerator for up to 1 week.

# LENTIL TACOS

**DF | GF | NF | V | 30 | OP**

½ packet taco seasoning

3 tablespoons water, plus more as needed

1 tablespoon avocado oil

1 teaspoon minced garlic

2 cups cooked brown lentils

6 corn or flour tortillas

2 avocados, pitted, peeled, and sliced

2 cups shredded romaine lettuce

2 tomatoes, finely chopped, or store-bought pico de gallo

Shredded cheese, for topping (optional)

In a small bowl, whisk together the taco seasoning and water.

Heat the oil in a large skillet over medium heat. Add the garlic and sauté for 1 minute. Add the lentils and taco seasoning mixture. Reduce the heat to low and simmer for 3 to 4 minutes, adding additional water if needed to prevent the lentils from drying out. The lentils should be very tender and very easy to mash with a fork.

Warm up each tortilla in a skillet over low heat for about 30 seconds on each side.

Spoon the lentil mixture into the tortillas, then top with the avocado, romaine, tomato, and cheese (if using). Serve.

---

**COOKING TIP:** If you can't find precooked lentils at your local grocery store or Trader Joe's, you can cook them yourself. Combine 1 cup uncooked lentils and 3 cups water or vegetable broth in a large saucepan. Bring to a boil over medium-high heat, then reduce the heat, cover the pan, and simmer until tender, 20 to 25 minutes.

**SERVING TIP:** Pair these tacos with a side of tortilla chips and Cashew Queso (see page 192).

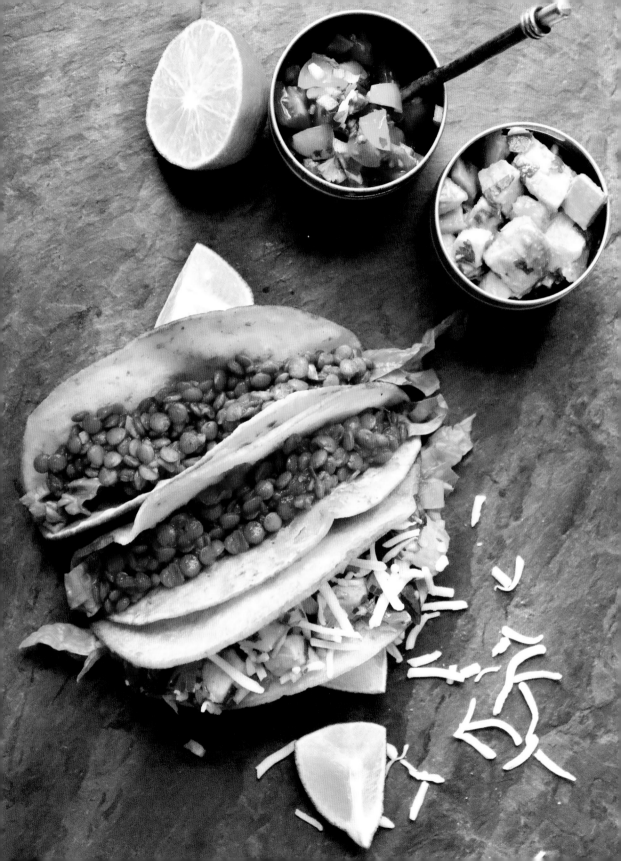

# CHIMICHURRI MUSHROOM TACOS

**DF | GF | NF | V**

**MAKES 4 SERVINGS**

Juice of 1 lime

¼ teaspoon smoked paprika

¼ teaspoon ground cumin

¼ teaspoon chili powder

⅛ teaspoon sea salt

2 tablespoons extra-virgin olive oil, divided

3 large portobello mushrooms, stemmed and sliced

½ medium yellow onion, sliced

8 small corn or flour tortillas

Chimichurri Sauce (recipe follows), for serving

In a large bowl or resealable plastic bag, combine the lime juice, paprika, cumin, chili powder, salt, and 1 tablespoon of the oil. Add the mushrooms and onion and toss to coat. Set aside to marinate for 30 minutes.

Heat the remaining 1 tablespoon of oil in a large skillet over medium heat. Add the marinated vegetables and cook, stirring occasionally, until the onion is translucent and the mushrooms are completely browned, about 8 minutes. Remove from the heat.

Warm each tortilla in a skillet over low heat for about 30 seconds on each side.

Fill each tortilla with a scoop of the mushroom mixture and top with a heaping spoonful of chimichurri. Serve.

---

**PERFORMANCE TIP:** If you'd like to make this dish higher in protein, you can add chicken or steak; to keep it vegan, add tempeh or tofu.

## CHIMICHURRI SAUCE

DF | GF | NF | V | 30 | NK | OP

MAKES 2 CUPS

1 cup loosely packed finely chopped fresh parsley

1 cup loosely packed finely chopped fresh cilantro

1 tablespoon minced garlic

⅓ cup extra-virgin olive oil

¼ cup red wine vinegar

1 teaspoon sea salt

1 teaspoon red pepper flakes

Combine all the ingredients in a small bowl and mix well. Store leftovers in an airtight container in the refrigerator for up to 2 weeks.

# FISH TACOS WITH PINEAPPLE-MANGO SALSA

**DF | GF | NF**

**2 tablespoons extra-virgin olive oil, avocado oil, or melted coconut oil**

**Juice of 1 lime**

**2 teaspoons chili powder**

**1 teaspoon garlic powder**

**1 teaspoon sweet paprika**

**1 teaspoon sea salt**

**½ teaspoon black pepper**

**1 pound fresh or thawed frozen cod fillets (or other white fish)**

**8 corn or small flour tortillas**

**Pineapple-Mango Salsa (recipe follows), for serving**

**Avocado slices, for serving**

**Lime wedges, for serving**

In a small bowl, whisk together the oil, lime juice, chili powder, garlic powder, paprika, salt, and pepper. Transfer the marinade to a large resealable plastic bag. Add the fish, seal the bag, and marinate in the refrigerator for 20 minutes.

Preheat the oven to 400°F.

Transfer the fish to a baking dish and bake for 10 to 12 minutes, until the fish flakes easily with a fork. Use the fork to break up the fish into small chunks.

Warm each tortilla in a skillet over low heat for about 30 seconds on each side.

Fill each tortilla with some fish, salsa, and avocado. Serve with lime wedges for squeezing.

---

## PINEAPPLE-MANGO SALSA

**DF | GF | NF | V | 30 | NK | OP**

MAKES 2½ CUPS

**1 mango, pitted, peeled, and finely chopped**

**1 cup finely chopped pineapple**

**½ jalapeño, seeded and minced**

**½ cup finely chopped fresh cilantro**

**Juice of ½ lemon**

**¼ teaspoon sea salt**

**¼ teaspoon black pepper**

In a medium bowl, combine all the ingredients and toss to mix well. Keep refrigerated in an airtight container until ready to use.

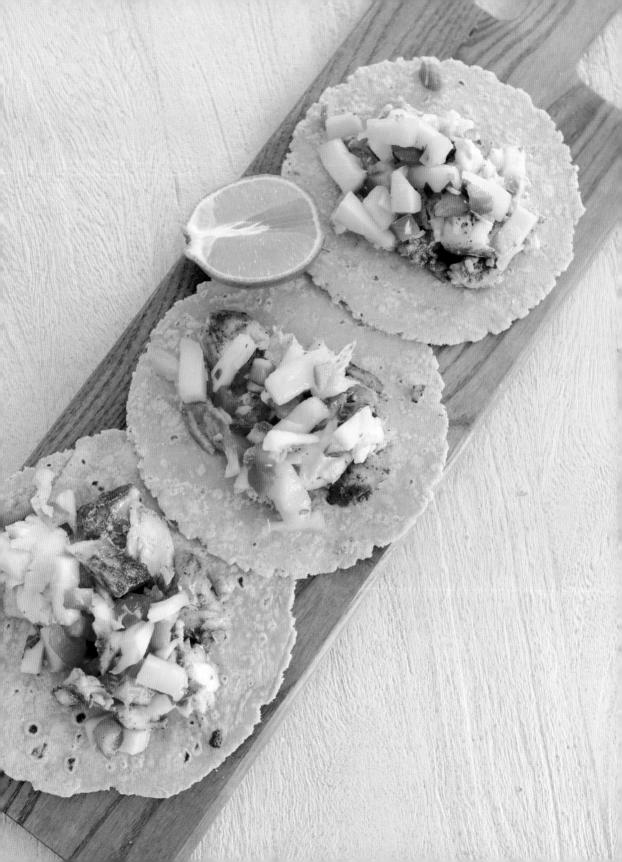

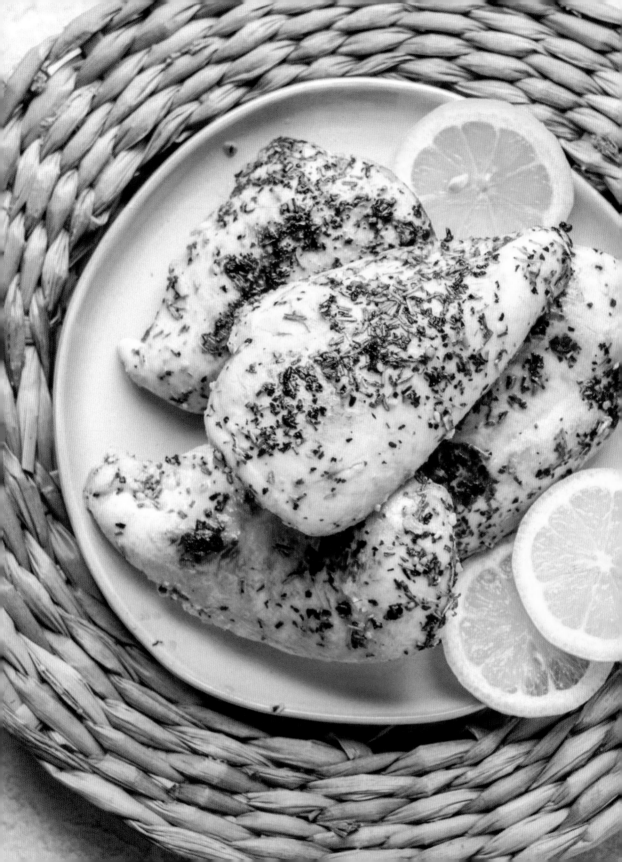

# CHAPTER EIGHT

# MAINS

When I was developing and perfecting the recipes for this book, I had several goals I mind. First and foremost, I wanted them to be nutritious and still taste delicious. Taste testing is such a fun job; it's safe to say I enjoy every minute of it! It was also very important to me to include a variety of cuisines, as well as a variety of dishes from plant-based to seafood and poultry. I realize that some weeknights you may be very limited on time and want something quick and convenient, like a quick stir-fry, marinated chicken, or simple baked salmon. Other nights, you may have more time to spend improving your skills in the kitchen or cooking for a crowd, in which you might want to try my Mexican-inspired chicken casserole, tempeh Bolognese, or homemade pizza. If you're a meat eater completely new to plant-based recipes, I recommend trying the tofu scramble or the pad thai. This is the chapter I am most excited for you to dig into—and return to week after week.

# TOFU PARMESAN

**NF | VEG | 30**

MAKES 3 SERVINGS

1 (15-ounce) package extra-firm tofu

1 large egg

3 tablespoons unsweetened nondairy milk or 2% milk

¼ cup whole-wheat breadcrumbs

2 tablespoons grated parmesan cheese

½ teaspoon dried basil

½ teaspoon dried oregano

¼ teaspoon garlic powder

Pinch of sea salt

1 cup marinara sauce

1–2 tablespoons extra-virgin olive oil

Shredded mozzarella, for topping (optional)

To press the tofu, wrap it in a clean dish towel or paper towels and place something heavy (such as a cast-iron skillet) on top. Let it drain for 15 minutes. (Pressing helps remove moisture from the tofu, allowing it to soak up more flavor.) After pressing, unwrap the tofu and cut it into 8 squares.

Whisk the egg and milk together in a small bowl. In a separate bowl, combine the breadcrumbs, parmesan, basil, oregano, garlic powder, and salt.

Dip each piece of tofu in the egg-milk mixture, then in the breadcrumb mixture until lightly coated.

Warm the marinara sauce in a small saucepan over low heat.

Heat 1 tablespoon of the oil in a large skillet over medium-high heat. Add the tofu in a single layer (depending on the size of your skillet, you may have to cook in batches). Cook the tofu until golden brown, about 4 minutes, then flip and cook until golden brown on the other side, 4 to 5 minutes. Transfer to a plate and repeat with the remaining oil and tofu if necessary.

Top each piece of tofu with a spoonful of warm marinara and shredded mozzarella (if using) and serve.

---

**COOKING TIP:** To make this vegan, swap the grated parmesan for nutritional yeast, and swap the egg-milk mixture for olive oil.

**SERVING TIP:** Serve with zucchini noodles, spaghetti squash, or whole-grain pasta and steamed veggies.

# TOFU SCRAMBLE

DF | GF | NF | V | 30

**MAKES 3 SERVINGS**

1 (15-ounce) package extra-firm tofu

2 tablespoons plus 1 teaspoon extra-virgin olive oil or avocado oil, divided

2 cups frozen hash browns (no need to thaw)

1 green bell pepper, seeded and chopped

1 red bell pepper, seeded and chopped

½ small white onion, chopped

2 tablespoons nutritional yeast

1½ teaspoons chili powder

1 teaspoon ground cumin

½ teaspoon garlic powder

¼ teaspoon sea salt

¼ teaspoon black pepper

3–4 tablespoons water

6 small corn or flour tortillas (optional)

Avocado slices, salsa, and fresh cilantro, for topping

To press the tofu, wrap it in a clean dish towel or paper towels and place something heavy (such as a cast-iron skillet) on top. Let it drain for 15 minutes. (Pressing helps remove moisture from the tofu, allowing it to soak up more flavor.)

Meanwhile, heat 2 tablespoons of the oil in a large skillet over medium-high heat. Add the hash browns, green pepper, red pepper, and onion and cook until the hash browns are golden brown and crisp, 7 to 8 minutes; set aside.

Combine the nutritional yeast, chili powder, cumin, garlic powder, salt, and pepper in a small bowl. Stir in enough of the water so that it becomes a pourable sauce, about 3 to 4 tablespoons.

Heat the remaining 1 teaspoon of oil in another skillet over medium heat. Unwrap the tofu and crumble it into bite-size pieces into the skillet. Sauté for 5 minutes, then pour in the sauce. Stir to make sure the sauce evenly coats the tofu and cook for another 4 to 5 minutes, until the tofu is lightly browned. Combine the tofu with the hash browns.

If using tortillas, warm up each tortilla in a skillet over low heat for about 30 seconds on each side. Spoon the mixture into the tortillas or onto plates. Top with avocado, salsa, and cilantro and serve.

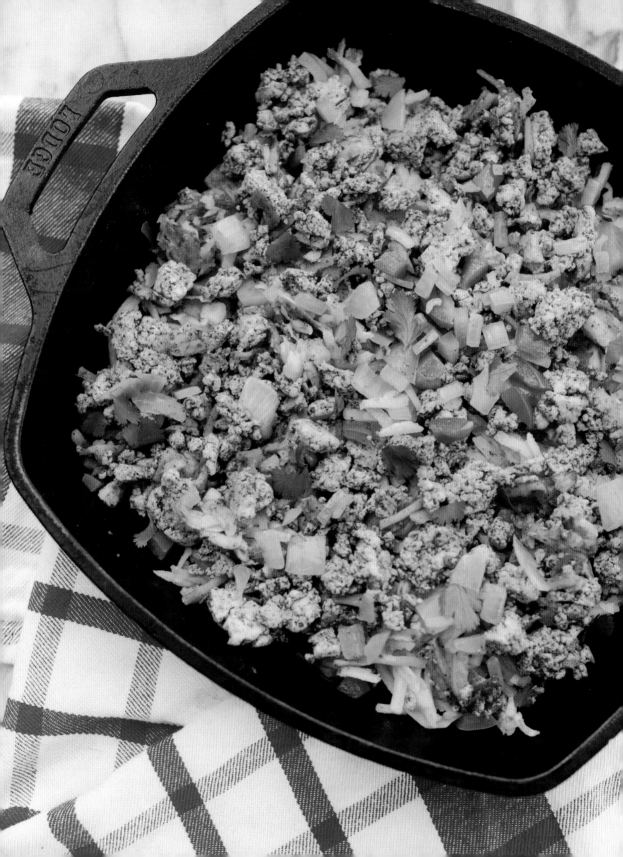

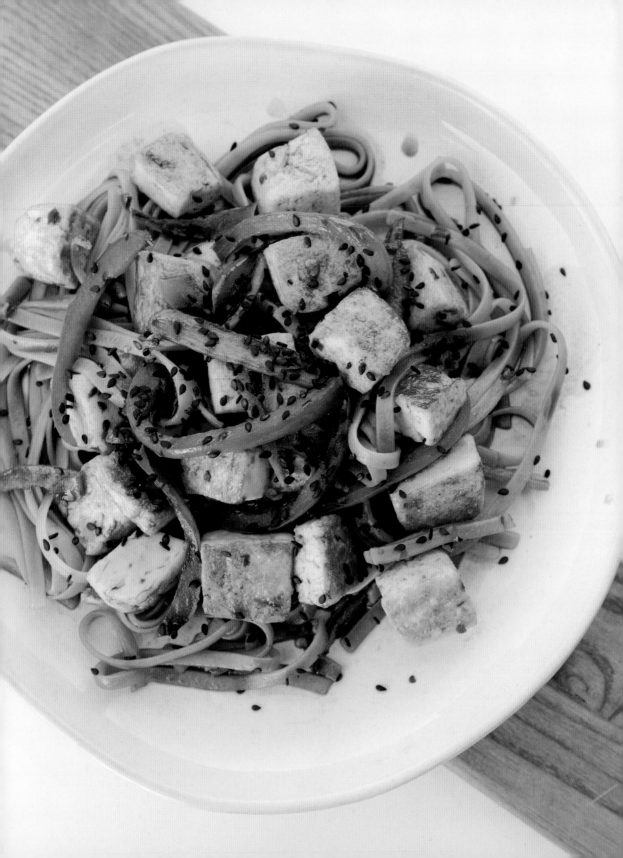

# SPICY PAD THAI WITH TOFU

**DF | GF | V | 30**

MAKES 4 SERVINGS

*Tofu and noodles*

**1 (15-ounce) package extra-firm tofu**

**8 ounces pad thai rice noodles**

*Sauce*

**¼ cup tamari or coconut aminos**

**3 tablespoons water**

**2 tablespoons peanut butter**

**2 teaspoons chile paste, or more to taste**

**2 teaspoons toasted sesame oil**

**2 teaspoons coconut sugar or brown sugar**

**1 teaspoon rice vinegar**

**1 teaspoon minced garlic**

*Stir-Fry*

**2 teaspoons toasted sesame oil or avocado oil, divided**

**1 tablespoon tamari or coconut aminos**

**1 cup shredded carrots**

**1 red bell pepper, seeded and chopped**

**6 shiitake mushrooms, sliced**

**½ medium white onion, chopped**

**Sesame seeds, for serving (optional)**

To press the tofu, wrap it in a clean dish towel or paper towels and place something heavy (such as a cast-iron skillet) on top. Let it drain for 15 minutes. (Pressing helps remove moisture from the tofu, allowing it to soak up more flavor.)

Meanwhile, cook the noodles according to the package directions and drain.

In a small bowl, whisk together the tamari, water, peanut butter, chile paste, oil, sugar, vinegar, and garlic to make the sauce; set aside.

Unwrap the tofu and cut it into bite-size pieces. Heat 1 teaspoon of the oil in a large skillet or wok over medium-high heat. Add the tofu and stir-fry until lightly browned, 5 to 7 minutes. Add the tamari and cook for 1 to 2 more minutes. Transfer the tofu to a plate.

Add the remaining 1 teaspoon of oil to the skillet, along with the carrots, bell pepper, mushrooms, and onion, and stir-fry for 5 minutes. Return the tofu to the skillet, pour in half of the sauce, and stir until well combined.

Add the cooked noodles and remaining sauce and stir until combined. Sprinkle with sesame seeds (if using) and serve immediately.

---

**COOKING TIP:** If you'd like your tofu to be even firmer in this recipe, try baking it first. This helps remove even more moisture and prevents it from crumbling. After pressing the tofu for 15 minutes, cut it into pieces and place on a baking sheet lined with parchment paper. Bake at 400°F for 20 minutes. Continue with the recipe as written.

# TEMPEH BOLOGNESE

DF | NF | V | 30

MAKES 4 SERVINGS

1 (8-ounce) package tempeh

1 tablespoon extra-virgin olive oil

1½ teaspoons minced garlic

½ cup finely chopped white onion

2 stalks celery, finely chopped

2 large carrots, finely chopped

½ cup finely chopped cremini mushrooms

1 (28-ounce) can crushed tomatoes

⅓ cup dry red wine

1 teaspoon dried basil

1 teaspoon dried oregano

1 teaspoon dried parsley

¼ teaspoon sea salt

8 ounces whole-grain pasta (spaghetti, penne, or angel hair), zucchini noodles, or spaghetti squash

Grated parmesan cheese or vegan cheese and fresh basil leaves, for topping (optional)

Use your hands or a cheese grater to crumble the tempeh into small pieces.

Heat the oil in a large skillet over medium-high heat. Add the garlic and onion and cook for 5 minutes, or until the onion is translucent. Reduce the heat to medium and add the crumbled tempeh, celery, carrots, and mushrooms. Cook for 5 minutes, then add the tomatoes, wine, basil, oregano, parsley, and salt, stirring to combine.

Simmer for 10 minutes, or until the liquid is slightly reduced. If the sauce becomes too thick, stir in a few tablespoons of water.

Meanwhile, bring a large pot of salted water to a boil over high heat. Add the pasta and cook according to the package directions until just tender. Drain and portion onto serving plates.

Spoon the sauce over the pasta, top with parmesan and/or basil (if using), and serve.

---

COOKING TIP: To make your own vegan parmesan cheese, combine ½ cup raw cashews, 2 tablespoons nutritional yeast, 1 teaspoon extra-virgin olive oil, ¼ teaspoon garlic powder, and ¼ teaspoon salt in a food processor. Pulse until the mixture becomes crumbly and resembles the texture of grated parmesan. Taste and add more seasonings if needed. Store in an airtight container in the refrigerator for up to 2 weeks.

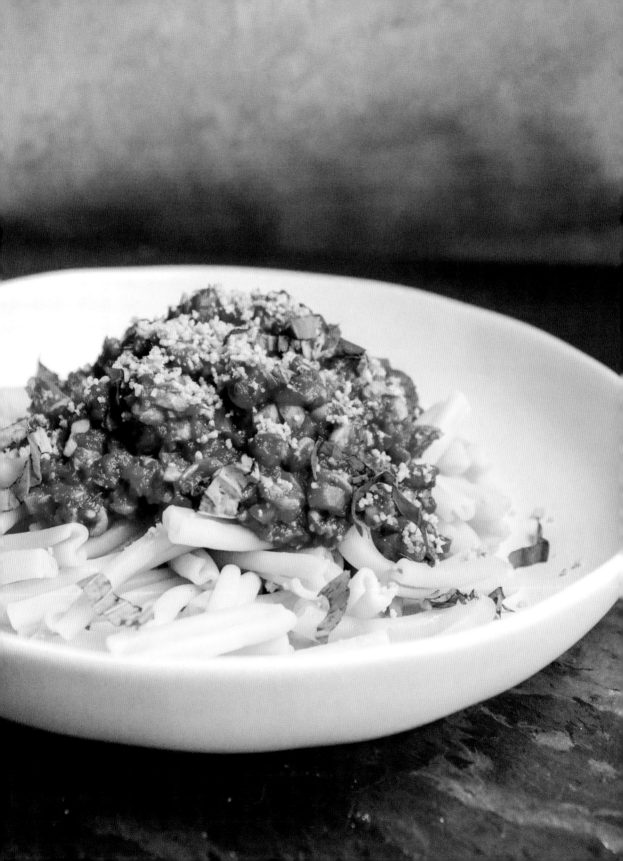

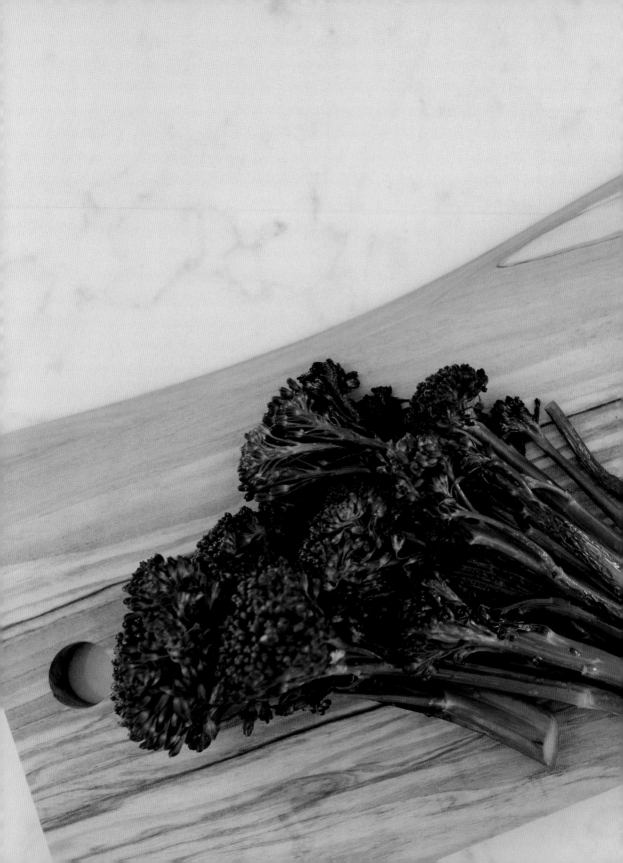

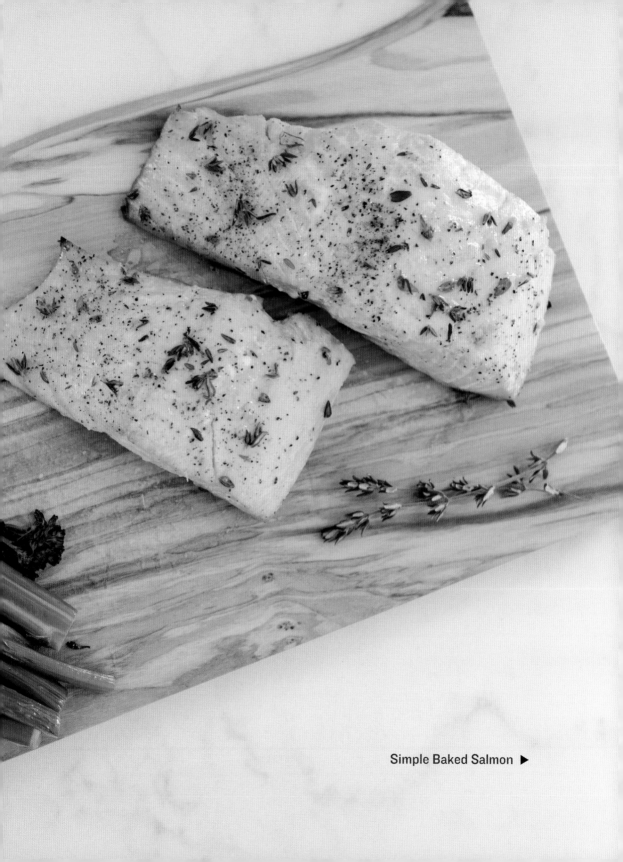

Simple Baked Salmon ▶

# SIMPLE BAKED SALMON

**DF | GF | NF | 30**

MAKES 3 SERVINGS

1 (1-pound) wild-caught salmon fillet, cut into 3 portions

3 tablespoons honey

1½ teaspoons freshly squeezed lemon juice

1½ teaspoons extra-virgin olive oil

1½ teaspoons white balsamic vinegar

1 tablespoon chopped fresh thyme or 1 teaspoon dried thyme

½ teaspoon minced garlic

¼ teaspoon sea salt

¼ teaspoon black pepper

Preheat the oven to 400°F. Lightly coat three 12-inch squares of aluminum foil with olive oil cooking spray.

Place a piece of salmon, skin-side down, in the center of each piece of foil. Fold the sides of the foil up over the salmon, creating a boat shape but leaving the top open.

Whisk together the honey, lemon juice, oil, vinegar, thyme, garlic, salt, and pepper in a small bowl. Pour the herb mixture evenly into each foil packet. Tightly close up the foil packets.

Bake for 12 to 15 minutes, until the salmon is cooked through and flakes easily with a fork. Open each packet carefully and serve the salmon with the accumulated juices.

---

**COOKING TIP:** If you purchase salmon with the skin still on, it is much easier to remove the skin after cooking. Simply slide a spatula between the salmon flesh and skin. You can also keep the skin on, if you prefer.

**SERVING TIP:** Pair this salmon with rice and steamed green beans, broccolini, or asparagus.

# ONE-PAN SALMON AND ROASTED VEGETABLES

DF | GF | NF | 30

2 cups fresh or frozen chopped vegetables

4 teaspoons extra-virgin olive oil, divided

1 tablespoon seasoning blend (such as Trader Joe's 21 Seasoning Salute)

2 tablespoons Dijon mustard

2 tablespoons honey

Juice of ½ lemon

1 teaspoon minced garlic

Sea salt and black pepper, to taste

1 (1-pound) wild-caught salmon fillet, cut into 3 portions

Preheat the oven to 400°F. Line a rimmed baking sheet with aluminum foil or parchment paper.

Spread out the vegetables in a single layer on the prepared baking sheet. Drizzle lightly with 2 teaspoons of the oil and sprinkle on the seasoning, tossing to coat the vegetables. Roast for 10 minutes.

In a small bowl, whisk together the mustard, the honey, the lemon juice, the remaining 2 teaspoons of oil, and the garlic. Brush onto the tops and sides of the salmon pieces. Season with salt and pepper.

Move the roasted vegetables to the sides of the baking sheet to make room for the salmon fillets in the center. Place the salmon between the vegetables.

Roast for 13 to 14 minutes, or until the salmon flakes easily with a fork. Serve the salmon with the vegetables.

---

**SERVING TIP:** Pair this with a side of rice or quinoa.

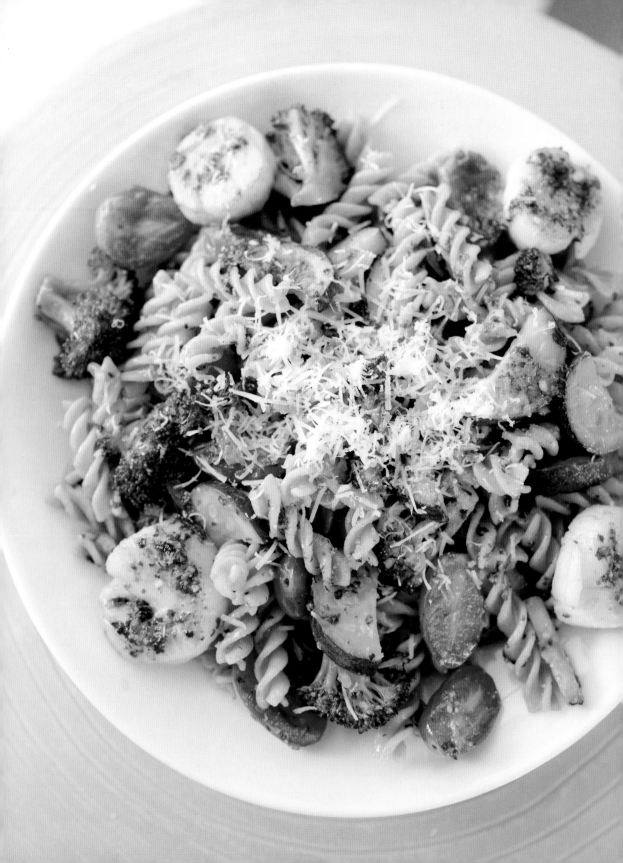

# WHOLE-GRAIN PESTO FUSILLI WITH SCALLOPS

30

8 ounces whole-grain fusilli

1 tablespoon plus
1 teaspoon extra-virgin
olive oil or butter, divided

1 zucchini, sliced

½ cup cherry tomatoes

2 cups chopped broccoli
florets

1 pound scallops or
uncooked shrimp, peeled
and deveined

Juice of ½ lemon

⅛ teaspoon sea salt

⅛ teaspoon black pepper

⅓ cup Basil Pesto (recipe
follows) or store-bought
pesto

Grated parmesan cheese,
for topping (optional)

Bring a large pot of salted water to a boil over high heat. Add the pasta and cook according to the package directions until just tender. Drain and set aside.

Meanwhile, heat 1 teaspoon of the oil in a large skillet over medium-high heat. Add the zucchini, tomatoes, and broccoli and sauté for 5 to 7 minutes, until tender. Transfer the vegetables to a plate. Add the remaining 1 tablespoon of oil to the skillet, then add the scallops, lemon juice, salt, and pepper. Cook the scallops until both sides are lightly browned, about 2 minutes per side.

Combine the pasta, vegetables, and pesto in a serving bowl, stirring to combine. Place the scallops on top of pasta with a bit of pesto on each. Top with grated parmesan (if using) and serve.

---

## BASIL PESTO

GF | VEG | 30

MAKES ½ CUP

2 cups fresh basil
leaves

2 cloves garlic

¼ cup pine nuts

1 tablespoon water

3 tablespoons grated
parmesan cheese

Sea salt and black
pepper, to taste

3 tablespoons extra-
virgin olive oil

Combine the basil, garlic, pine nuts, water, parmesan, salt, and pepper in a food processor or blender. Pulse until smooth, then drizzle in the oil through the feed tube while still pulsing. The pesto should be thick, not runny. Store in an airtight container in the refrigerator for up to 1 week.

# SHRIMP AND BROCCOLI STIR-FRY

DF | GF | NF

2 tablespoons honey

1½ tablespoons tamari or coconut aminos

1 (1-inch) piece fresh ginger, minced

½ teaspoon minced garlic

½ pound uncooked shrimp, peeled and deveined

1 cup fresh or frozen broccoli

Pinch of salt

1 tablespoon toasted sesame oil or extra-virgin olive oil

1½ cups cooked brown or jasmine rice

Sesame seeds and chopped scallions, for serving

In a small bowl, whisk together the honey, tamari, ginger, and garlic. Pour half of the mixture into a large resealable plastic bag or bowl. Add the shrimp, seal the bag or cover the bowl, and refrigerate for 20 minutes. Reserve the rest of the mixture to use as a stir-fry sauce.

Meanwhile, pour ¼ inch of water into a saucepan and bring to a boil over medium-high heat. Add the broccoli and salt. Reduce the heat to medium, cover, and steam the broccoli for 5 to 7 minutes, until bright green and fork-tender. Drain.

In a large skillet or wok, heat the oil over medium-high heat. Add the marinated shrimp and sear for 1 to 2 minutes on each side. Reduce the heat to low. Add the steamed broccoli and reserved sauce. Stir until well combined, 2 to 3 minutes.

Top the rice with the shrimp and broccoli, garnish with sesame seeds and chopped scallions, and serve.

COOKING TIP: Frozen organic brown rice or jasmine rice makes a great option when you're short on time. It can be prepared in just a few minutes in a microwave or in a skillet on the stovetop.

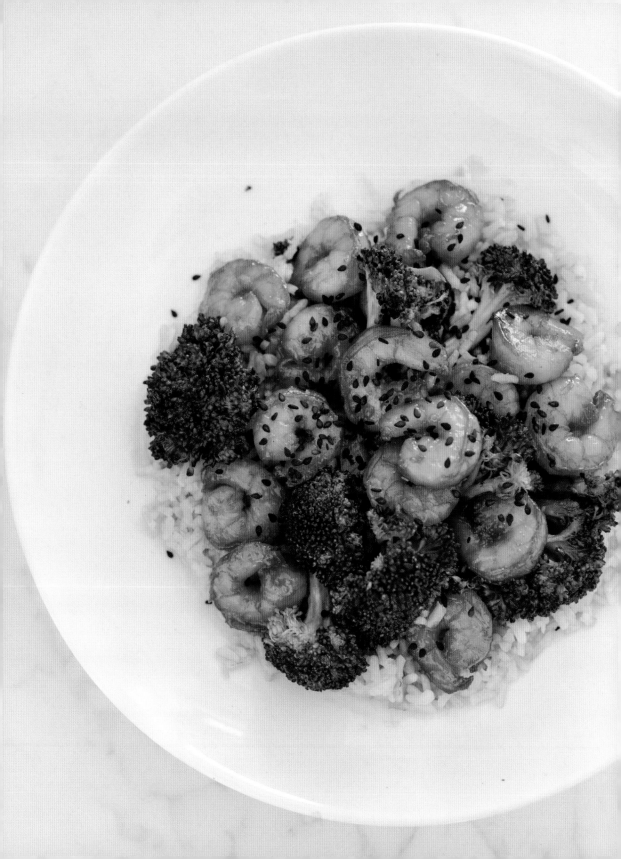

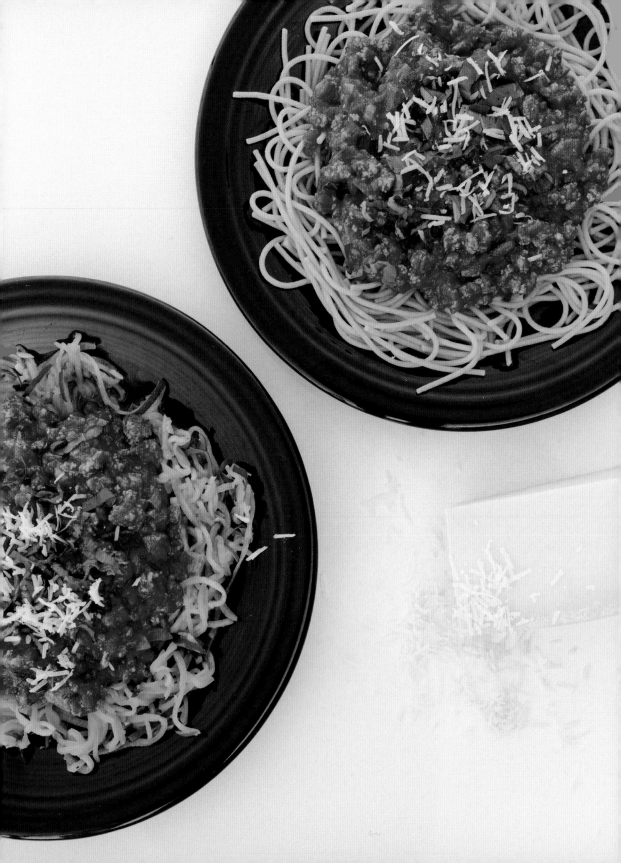

# TURKEY BOLOGNESE

**DF | GF | NF**

3 tablespoons extra-virgin olive oil, divided

½ cup chopped white onion

1½ teaspoons minced garlic

1½ pounds lean ground turkey

1 (28-ounce) can crushed tomatoes

⅓ cup loosely packed chopped fresh basil

1 teaspoon dried oregano

1 teaspoon dried parsley

¼ teaspoon sea salt

¼ teaspoon black pepper

3 large zucchini

Grated or shaved parmesan cheese, for garnish (optional)

Heat 1 tablespoon of the oil in a large skillet over medium-high heat. Add the onion and garlic and sauté for about 5 minutes, or until the onion is translucent.

Add the turkey and cook, breaking it up into small pieces with a spoon, for 8 to 10 minutes, until no longer pink. Add the tomatoes, basil, oregano, parsley, salt, and pepper, stirring until everything is well combined. Bring to a boil, then reduce the heat to medium-low and simmer for about 15 minutes, until the sauce thickens.

Meanwhile, spiralize the zucchini with a spiralizer or thinly slice them with a mandoline. Heat the remaining 2 tablespoons of oil in another skillet over medium-high heat. Add the zucchini noodles and cook, stirring frequently, for 3 to 4 minutes. Do not overcook; they will become soggy.

Divide the zucchini noodles among the serving plates. Top with the Bolognese, garnish with parmesan cheese (if using), and serve.

---

**PERFORMANCE TIP:** To increase the carbohydrates of this dish, add whole-grain spaghetti along with the zucchini noodles.

# TURKEY BURGERS

DF | NF | 30

1½ pounds lean
ground turkey

1 large egg

1 teaspoon minced garlic

2 tablespoons
Worcestershire sauce

1 tablespoon dried
parsley

Pinch of salt and black
pepper

2 tablespoons
avocado oil

In a large mixing bowl, combine the turkey, egg, garlic, Worcestershire sauce, parsley, salt, and pepper. Use your hands to form the meat mixture into 6 patties.

Heat the oil in a large skillet over medium heat. Add the patties and cook until just golden and cooked through, about 6 minutes per side. Serve.

---

**SERVING TIP:** These burgers pair great with Baked Potato Chips (see page 175) and a side salad or steamed vegetables.

# SLOW OR INSTANT TURKEY MEATBALLS

NF | NK

MAKES 6 SERVINGS

**1¼ pounds lean ground turkey**

**3 tablespoons finely chopped fresh parsley plus more for garnish (optional)**

**1 teaspoon dried basil**

**1 teaspoon minced garlic**

**1 large egg**

**¼ cup whole-wheat breadcrumbs**

**¼ cup grated parmesan cheese, plus more for garnish (optional)**

**Pinch of sea salt and black pepper**

**1 (25-ounce) jar marinara sauce**

Combine the turkey, parsley, basil, garlic, egg, breadcrumbs, parmesan, salt, and pepper in a large bowl. Using your hands, combine the meatball mixture. Form 24 even balls.

If using a **slow cooker**, pour the marinara sauce into the slow cooker. Place the meatballs in the sauce and use a small spoon to cover the top of each meatball with sauce. Cover and cook on high for 3 hours or on low for 6 hours, until cooked through.

If using a **pressure cooker**, pour the marinara sauce into the pressure cooker. Place the meatballs in the sauce and use a small spoon to cover the top of each meatball with sauce. Cover and turn the valve to the sealing position. Select the "meat cook" function. When the cooking time is up, let the pressure cooker naturally release pressure for 10 minutes, then flip the valve to the venting position.

Serve the meatballs garnished with fresh parsley and/or grated parmesan (if using).

---

**SERVING TIP:** Try the meatballs with whole-wheat spaghetti and a side of vegetables.

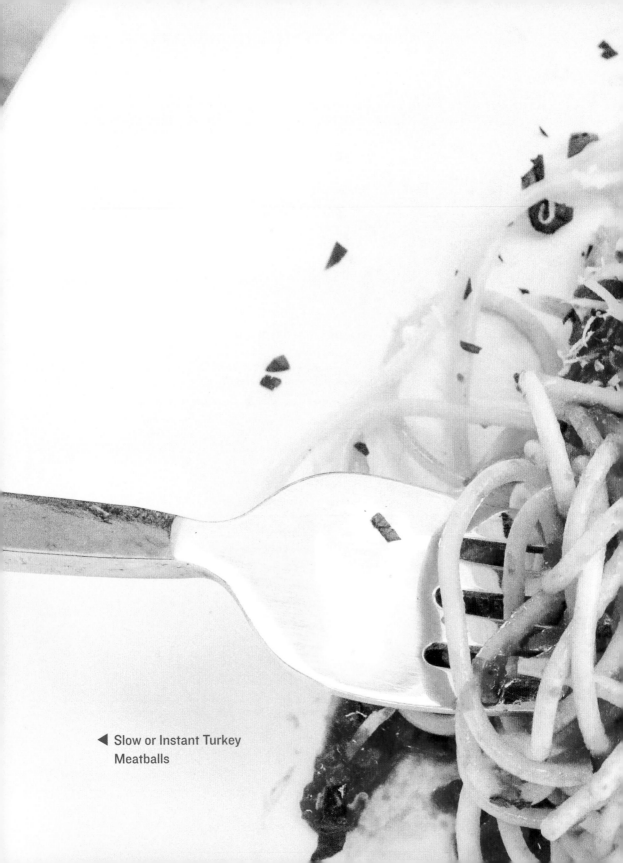

◀ Slow or Instant Turkey
Meatballs

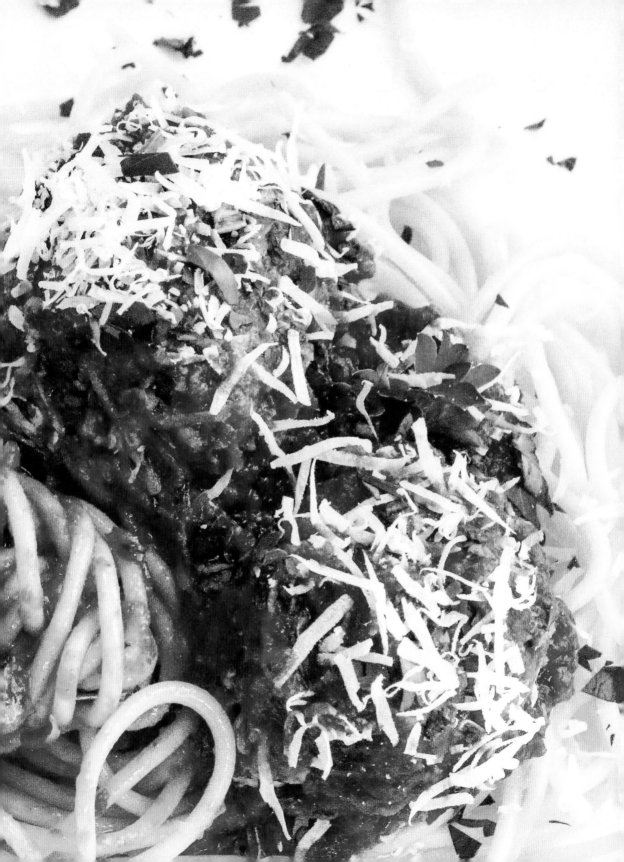

# CHICKEN MEATBALLS

**GF | 30**

**1 pound ground chicken breast**

**¼ cup almond flour or whole-wheat breadcrumbs**

**⅓ cup grated parmesan cheese**

**1 teaspoon minced garlic**

**1 large egg**

**1 tablespoon Italian seasoning**

**1 tablespoon dried parsley**

**½ teaspoon sea salt**

**½ teaspoon black pepper**

**1 cup marinara or alfredo sauce**

Preheat the oven to 425°F. Line a rimmed baking sheet with parchment paper or spray it lightly with olive oil cooking spray.

In a large mixing bowl, combine the chicken, almond flour, parmesan, garlic, egg, Italian seasoning, parsley, salt, and pepper. Use your hands to mix until well combined, then roll the mixture into 2-inch meatballs.

Arrange the meatballs on the prepared baking sheet and bake for 25 minutes, until cooked through.

Toss the meatballs with the marinara sauce and serve.

---

**COOKING TIP:** To make this recipe dairy-free, simply omit the parmesan.

**SERVING TIP:** Serve these meatballs with whole-wheat or brown rice pasta and vegetables.

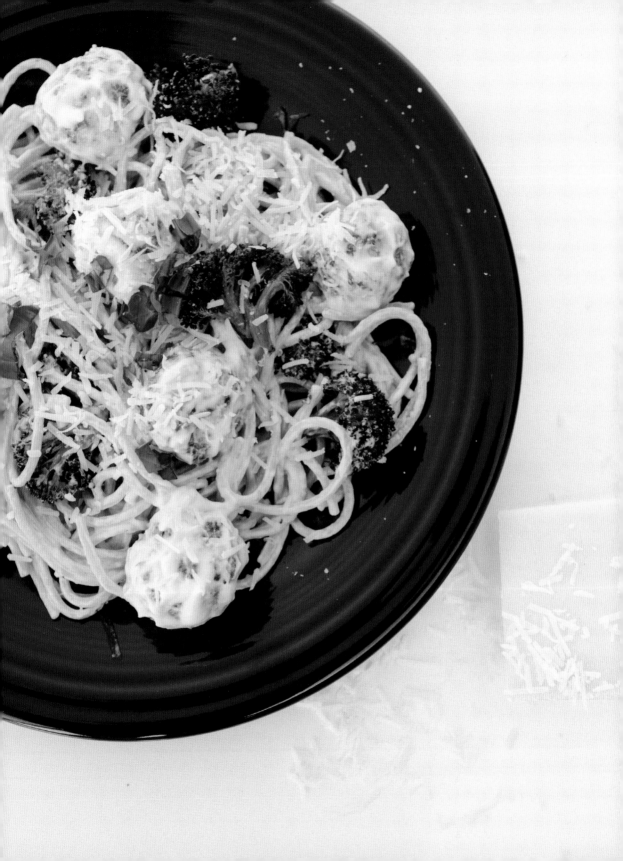

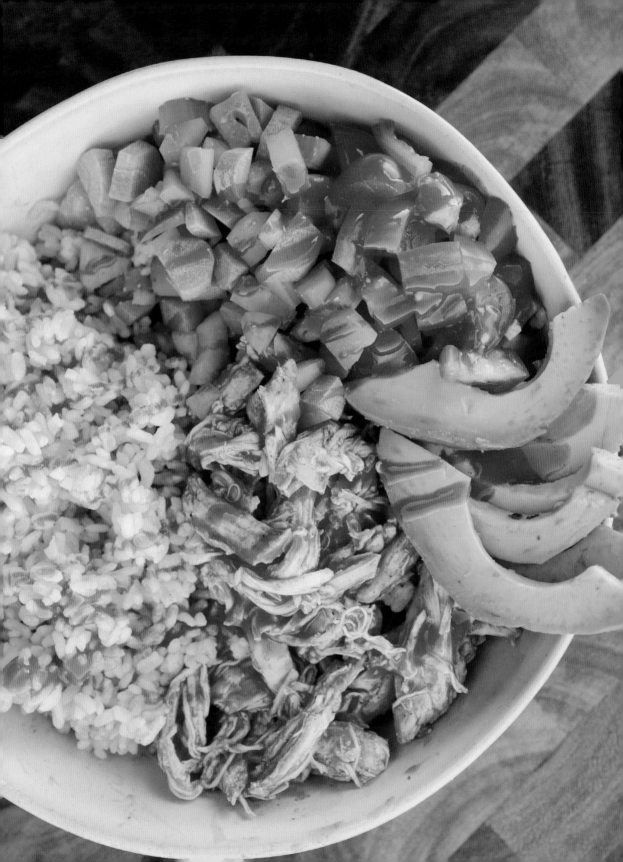

# SHREDDED BUFFALO CHICKEN

**DF | GF | NF | NK**

MAKES 8 SERVINGS

1½ cups buffalo sauce, such as The New Primal

3 tablespoons water

½ teaspoon garlic powder

½ teaspoon onion powder

½ teaspoon black pepper

2 pounds boneless, skinless chicken breasts

In a medium bowl, whisk together the buffalo sauce, water, garlic powder, onion powder, and pepper.

If using a **slow cooker**, put the chicken breasts in the slow cooker and cover them with the sauce mixture. Cover and cook on high for 3 to 4 hours or on low for 5 to 6 hours, until the chicken is cooked through.

If using a **pressure cooker,** put the chicken breasts in the pressure cooker and cover them with the sauce mixture. Cover and turn the valve to the sealing position. Select the "manual/pressure cook" function and set to 14 minutes. When the cooking time is up, let the pressure cooker naturally release pressure for 10 minutes, then flip the valve to the venting position.

Transfer the chicken to a cutting board. Use two forks to shred the chicken. Return it to the pot, and stir to combine. Serve.

---

**SERVING TIP:** This chicken is perfect in tacos (see page 122) or for topping a salad or rice bowl.

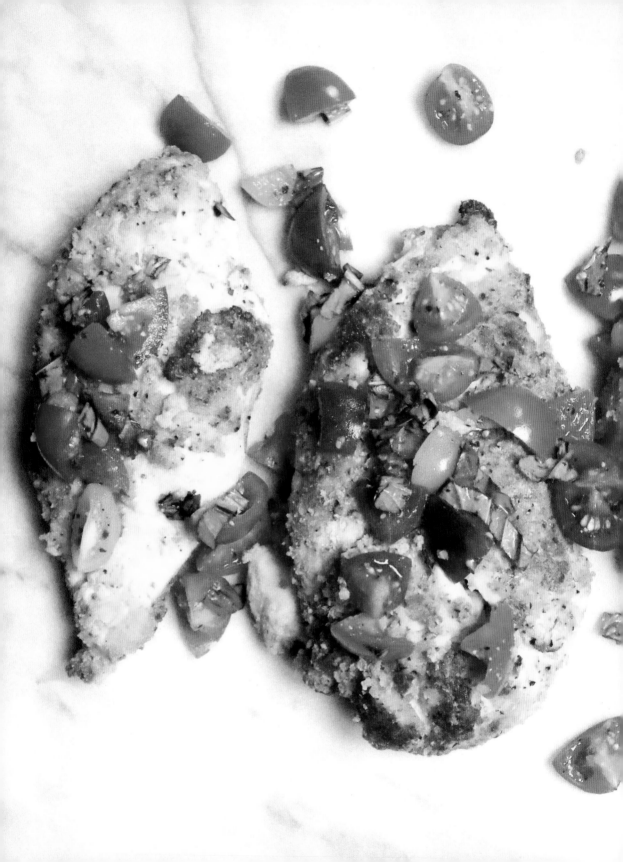

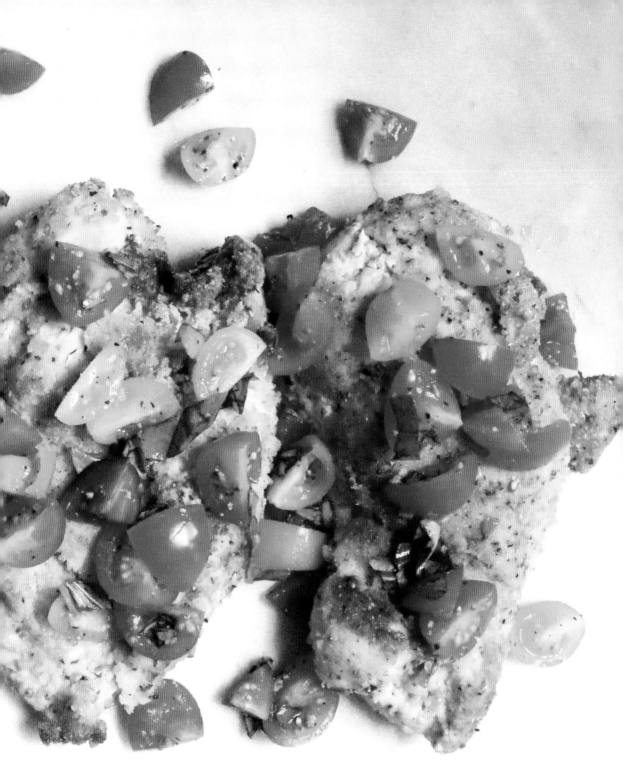

Bruschetta Chicken ▶

# BRUSCHETTA CHICKEN

**DF | NF | 30**

2 large egg whites

¼ cup unsweetened nondairy milk or 2% milk

½ cup whole-wheat breadcrumbs or almond flour

¾ teaspoon garlic powder, divided

¾ teaspoon black pepper, divided

½ teaspoon dried oregano

1½ pounds boneless, skinless chicken breasts

1 tablespoon extra-virgin olive oil

2 large tomatoes, chopped

¼ cup loosely packed chopped fresh basil

Pinch of sea salt

Preheat the oven to 375°F.

In a small bowl, whisk together the egg whites and milk. In a separate small bowl, mix together the breadcrumbs, ½ teaspoon of the garlic powder, ½ teaspoon of the pepper, and the oregano. Dip each chicken breast into the milk mixture, then coat in the breadcrumb mixture.

Heat the oil in a large oven-safe skillet (preferably cast-iron) over medium-high heat. Add the chicken and cook for 2 to 3 minutes on each side, until lightly browned.

Transfer the skillet to the oven and bake for 20 minutes, or until the chicken is golden brown and cooked through.

While the chicken is baking, combine the tomatoes, the basil, the salt, the remaining ¼ teaspoon of garlic powder, and the remaining ¼ teaspoon of pepper in a medium bowl. Refrigerate until the chicken is ready.

Top the chicken with the tomato mixture and serve.

---

**COOKING TIP:** If you don't have an oven-safe skillet, simply brown the chicken in any skillet and then transfer it to a lightly greased baking pan.

**SERVING TIP:** Try this with a side of quinoa, rice, or whole-wheat pasta and steamed vegetables.

# MEDITERRANEAN CHICKEN

**DF | GF | NF**

MAKES 4 SERVINGS

¼ cup extra-virgin olive oil

Juice of 1 lemon

1½ teaspoons minced garlic

1 tablespoon chopped fresh rosemary

1 tablespoon chopped fresh oregano

1 tablespoon chopped fresh thyme

¼ teaspoon sea salt

¼ teaspoon black pepper

1½ pounds boneless, skinless chicken breasts, cut into strips

Combine the oil, lemon juice, garlic, rosemary, oregano, thyme, salt, and pepper in a shallow bowl or casserole dish and stir until well combined. Place the chicken in the mixture and toss to coat. Cover and refrigerate for at least 2 hours or as long as overnight.

Heat a large skillet over medium-high heat. Add the chicken and cook for 4 minutes on each side, until fully cooked throughout. Serve.

**COOKING TIP:** If you do not have any fresh herbs available, you can always substitute with dried. Dried herbs are generally about three times as potent as fresh, so 1 tablespoon of fresh herbs can be replaced with 1 teaspoon dried.

**SERVING TIP:** This chicken can be used to make gyros (see page 125). It's also great on top of a salad, or it can be paired with a grain and vegetable for a simple dinner.

# THAI PEANUT CHICKEN

**DF | GF | 30**

*Peanut Sauce*

⅓ cup creamy natural peanut butter

2 tablespoons tamari or coconut aminos

1 tablespoon honey

1 tablespoon rice vinegar

1 teaspoon chile paste

½ teaspoon garlic powder

¼ teaspoon red pepper flakes, or more to taste

3–5 tablespoons water

*Chicken and Noodles*

1 tablespoon toasted sesame oil, plus more as needed

1 pound boneless, skinless chicken breasts, cut into bite-size pieces

1–2 cups frozen stir-fry mixed vegetables (bell peppers, snow peas, carrots, onions; no need to thaw)

8 ounces cooked brown rice Thai noodles, zucchini noodles, or brown rice

Chopped scallions, sesame seeds, or crushed peanuts, for serving

Combine the peanut butter, tamari, honey, vinegar, chile paste, garlic powder, and red pepper flakes in a food processor or blender. Process to combine. With the machine running, slowly add the water until the desired consistency is reached. Set aside.

Heat the oil in a large skillet over medium-high heat. Add the chicken and cook until no longer pink, 3 to 4 minutes on each side. Add the vegetables and a little more oil as needed. Cook for 5 to 7 minutes, until the chicken is fully cooked and the vegetables are tender.

Reduce the heat to low. Slowly pour in the peanut sauce, tossing to coat. Portion out the noodles and top with the chicken and vegetables. Garnish with scallions and serve.

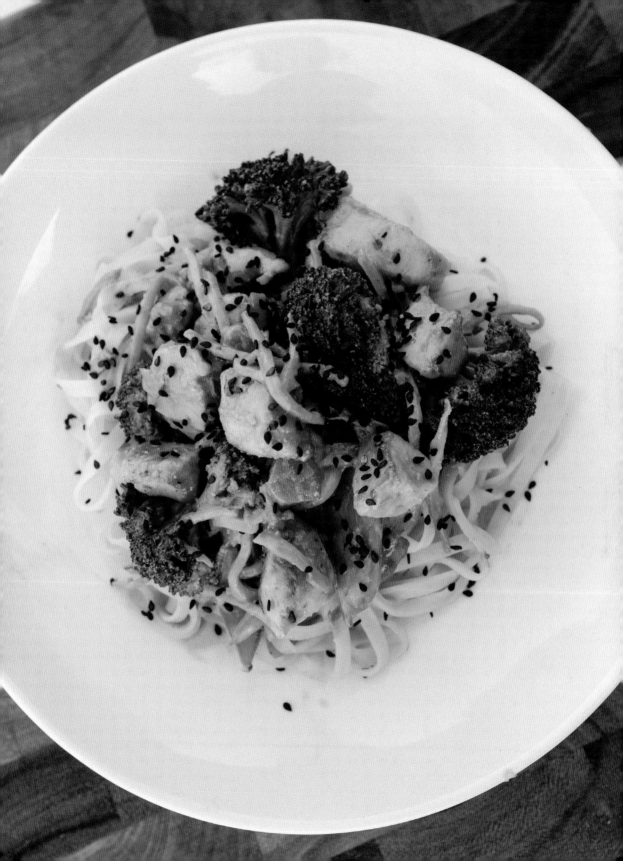

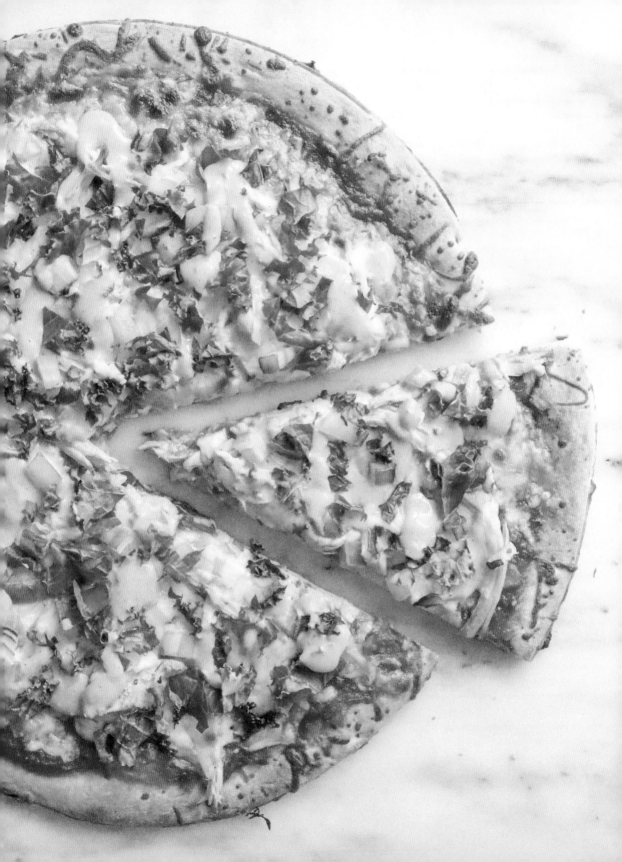

# BUFFALO CHICKEN PIZZA

NF

1 tablespoon extra-virgin olive oil

8 ounces boneless, skinless chicken breasts

Sea salt and black pepper, to taste

1 (12-inch) whole-wheat pizza crust

⅓ cup marinara sauce

½ cup shredded mozzarella cheese

2 tablespoons grated parmesan cheese

¾ cup shredded spinach or kale

¼ cup chopped red onion

1 tablespoon plain Greek yogurt

1 tablespoon buffalo sauce, such as The New Primal

Preheat the oven to 400°F to 450°F, or according to the pizza crust's package directions.

Heat the oil in a medium skillet over medium-high heat. Season the chicken with salt and pepper. Add the chicken to the skillet and cook for about 5 minutes, then flip and cook for another 4 to 5 minutes, until the chicken is cooked through. Transfer the chicken to a cutting board to cool slightly.

Using two forks, shred the chicken into very small pieces.

Place the pizza crust on a baking sheet (unless the package directions say to bake it directly on the oven rack). Spread the marinara sauce on the crust. Add the shredded chicken, mozzarella, parmesan, spinach, and onion.

Bake until the cheese is bubbly and brown, 12 to 15 minutes or according to the pizza crust's package directions.

Meanwhile, combine the yogurt and buffalo sauce in a small bowl. When the pizza is done, drizzle the sauce on top, cut the pizza into slices, and serve.

COOKING TIP: If you are short on time, use leftover Shredded Buffalo Chicken (see page 159) or a store-bought rotisserie chicken.

# PESTO BAKED CHICKEN

**GF | 30 | OP**

**4 (6-ounce) boneless, skinless chicken breasts**

**4 teaspoons Basil Pesto (page 147) or store-bought pesto**

**¼ cup shredded mozzarella cheese**

**3 Roma tomatoes, thinly sliced**

Preheat the oven to 400°F. Lightly spray a baking pan or casserole dish with olive oil cooking spray.

Place each chicken breast between two sheets of parchment paper and use a meat mallet or small, heavy skillet to pound the chicken breasts to an even 1-inch thickness. Place the chicken in a single layer in the prepared dish. Spread 1 teaspoon pesto on each chicken breast.

Bake for 15 minutes. Scatter the mozzarella and tomato slices on top of each chicken breast. Bake for another 5 minutes, or until the cheese is melted and the chicken is cooked through. Serve.

**COOKING TIP:** To make the recipe dairy-free, omit the mozzarella cheese on top of the chicken and the parmesan in the pesto. If you're short on time, use store-bought pesto, such as Trader Joe's vegan kale pesto.

**SERVING TIP:** Serve with a side of rice or whole-grain pasta and vegetables.

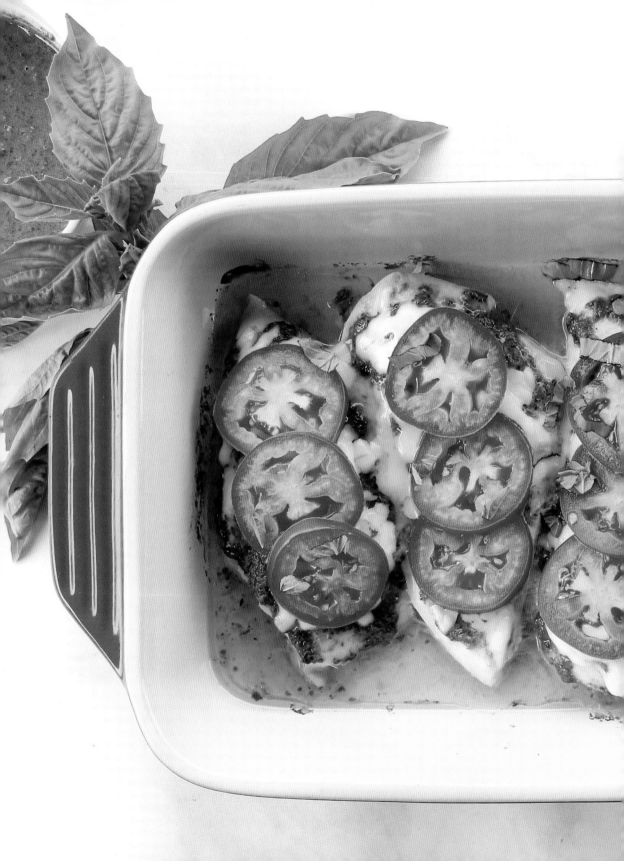

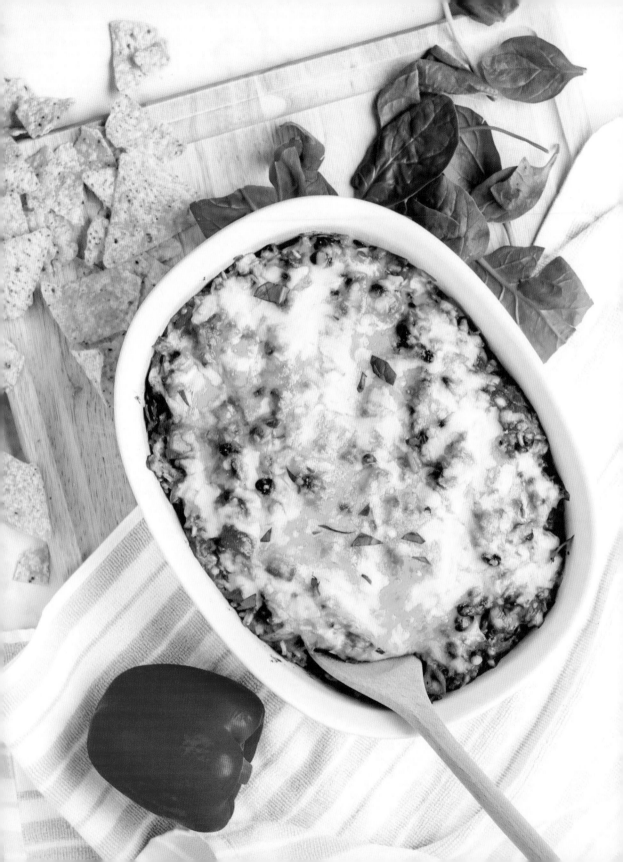

# MEXICAN-INSPIRED CHICKEN CASSEROLE

GF | NF

2 tablespoons extra-virgin olive oil or avocado oil

1 pound boneless, skinless chicken breasts, cut into bite-size pieces

1 teaspoon minced garlic

1 green bell pepper, seeded and chopped

1 medium white onion, chopped

2 tablespoons chili powder

1 teaspoon ground cumin

½ teaspoon sea salt

½ teaspoon black pepper

½ teaspoon cayenne pepper

2 cups frozen cooked brown rice or quinoa, reheated according to package directions

1 (15-ounce) can black beans, rinsed and drained

1 (15-ounce) can fire-roasted diced tomatoes, drained

½ cup chopped spinach or kale

1 cup plain Greek yogurt

½ cup shredded mozzarella cheese

½ cup shredded cheddar cheese

Preheat the oven to 350°F.

Heat the oil in a large pot over medium-high heat. Add the chicken and cook for 4 to 5 minutes on each side. Add the garlic, bell pepper, onion, chili powder, cumin, salt, black pepper, and cayenne and cook, stirring, for 3 to 5 minutes, until the bell pepper and onion are softened.

Add the rice, beans, diced tomatoes, and spinach. Reduce the heat to low and cook for 2 to 4 minutes, until heated through. Add the yogurt, half of the mozzarella, and half of the cheddar. Stir until well combined.

Transfer the mixture to a casserole dish. Sprinkle the remaining mozzarella and cheddar on top.

Bake for 15 to 20 minutes, until the cheese is slightly browned. Let cool for 5 to 10 minutes before serving.

---

**COOKING TIP:** To make this vegetarian, omit the chicken and use two cans of black beans.

# HONEY-GARLIC CHICKEN

DF | GF | NF | 30

MAKES 4 SERVINGS

2 large eggs

½ cup chickpea crumbs, brown rice flour, or whole-wheat breadcrumbs

1 pound boneless, skinless chicken breasts, cut into bite-size pieces

½ cup honey

2 tablespoons tamari or coconut aminos

2½ teaspoons minced garlic

1 tablespoon arrowroot or cornstarch

3 tablespoons water

1 tablespoon sesame seeds, for topping (optional)

Preheat the oven to 400°F. Line a rimmed baking sheet with parchment paper or aluminum foil.

Whisk the eggs in a small bowl. Put the chickpea crumbs in a separate small bowl. Dip each piece of chicken into the egg, then roll it in the breadcrumbs, coating lightly.

Transfer the coated chicken pieces to the prepared baking sheet in a single layer. Bake for 12 to 15 minutes, until the chicken is cooked through.

Meanwhile, combine the honey, tamari, and garlic in a large saucepan and heat over medium-high heat. In a small bowl, whisk together the arrowroot and water to make a slurry. Add the slurry to the saucepan and cook, stirring, for 3 to 4 minutes, until the sauce thickens.

Add the chicken to the saucepan and stir to coat each piece evenly. Sprinkle with the sesame seeds (if using) and serve.

COOKING TIP: There are several gluten-free alternatives to traditional breadcrumbs. Chickpea crumbs, such as Watusee brand, provide a crispier texture similar to panko breadcrumbs. Because brown rice flour and almond flour are much finer, they won't provide the same crispy texture but still serve as a good alternative.

SERVING TIP: Serve with rice and broccoli, tri-color cauliflower, or stir-fry vegetables.

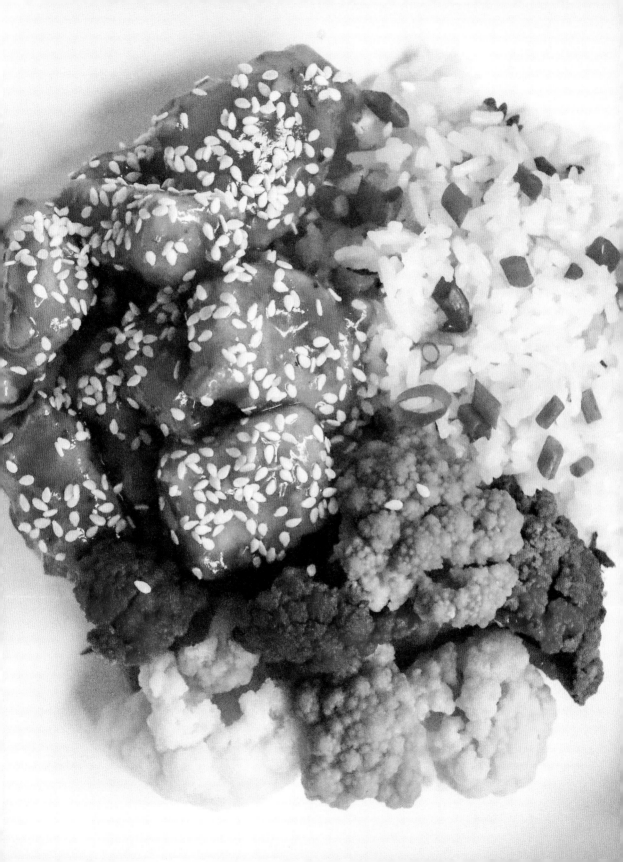

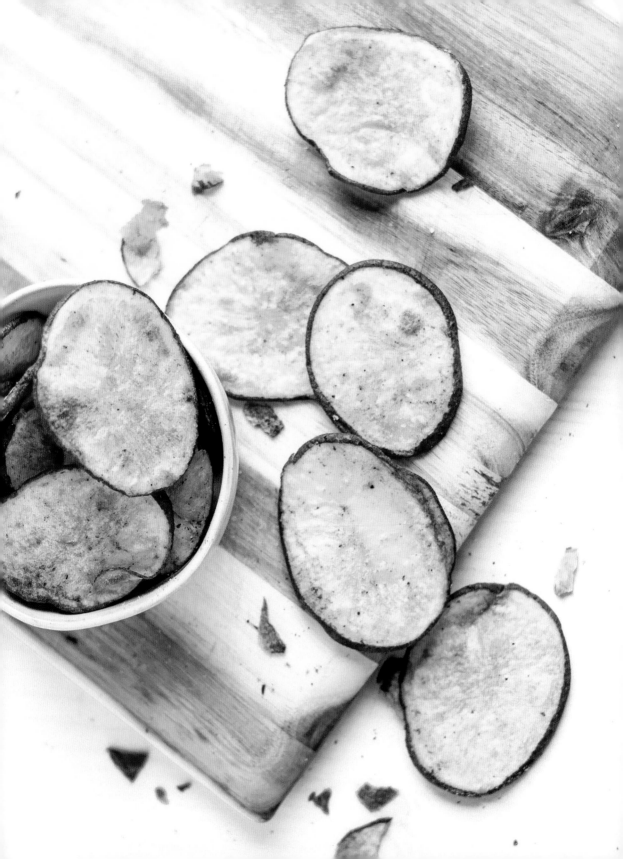

# ALMOND-CRUSTED CHICKEN WITH BAKED POTATO CHIPS

DF | GF

MAKES 4 SERVINGS

**1 pound boneless, skinless chicken breasts**

**¾ cup almond meal**

**1½ teaspoons garlic powder**

**1½ teaspoons onion powder**

**½ teaspoon dried basil**

**½ teaspoon sea salt**

**2 large eggs**

**Baked Potato Chips (recipe follows), for serving**

Preheat the oven to 425°F. Line a rimmed baking sheet with parchment paper or spray it generously with olive oil cooking spray.

Cut the chicken into thin strips.

In a small bowl, combine the almond meal, garlic powder, onion powder, basil, and salt and mix well. In a separate small bowl, whisk together the eggs.

Dip each chicken strip into the egg mixture, then roll it in the almond meal mixture, coating completely.

Arrange the chicken strips in a single layer on the prepared baking sheet. Bake for 15 minutes, flip each strip over, and bake for another 15 minutes, or until brown on both sides.

Serve with baked potato chips.

---

## BAKED POTATO CHIPS

DF | GF | NF | V | 30

MAKES 4 SERVINGS

**2 large russet potatoes**

**2 tablespoons avocado oil**

**1 teaspoon smoked paprika**

**½ teaspoon sea salt**

**½ teaspoon black pepper**

Preheat the oven to 425°F. Line a rimmed baking sheet with parchment paper and coat with a bit of avocado oil cooking spray.

Use a mandoline or chef's knife to cut the potatoes into very thin rounds. Put the potato rounds in a large mixing bowl. Add the oil, paprika, salt, and pepper and toss well to coat.

Arrange the potato chips in a single layer on the prepared baking sheet. Bake for 20 minutes, flip the potato chips, and bake for another 20 minutes, or until golden brown and crispy. Serve.

---

**COOKING TIP:** The chicken and potato chips bake at the same oven temperature, but the potato chips take a little longer, so you'll want to start them first.

# LEMON-GARLIC MARINATED CHICKEN

**DF | GF | NF**

MAKES 4 SERVINGS

**2 tablespoons avocado oil or extra-virgin olive oil**

**Juice of 1 lemon**

**1½ teaspoons minced garlic**

**1 tablespoon dried rosemary**

**1 tablespoon dried basil**

**Sea salt and black pepper, to taste**

**1½ pounds boneless, skinless chicken breasts**

In a small bowl, whisk together the oil, lemon juice, garlic, rosemary, basil, salt, and pepper. Transfer the marinade to a large resealable plastic bag. Add the chicken, seal the bag, and transfer to the refrigerator to marinate for at least 1 hour or as long as overnight.

Preheat the oven to 400°F.

Transfer the chicken to a casserole dish or baking pan and bake for 20 to 25 minutes, until the chicken is cooked through. Serve.

---

**SERVING TIP:** Serve with rice, quinoa, or potatoes and a side of steamed or roasted vegetables.

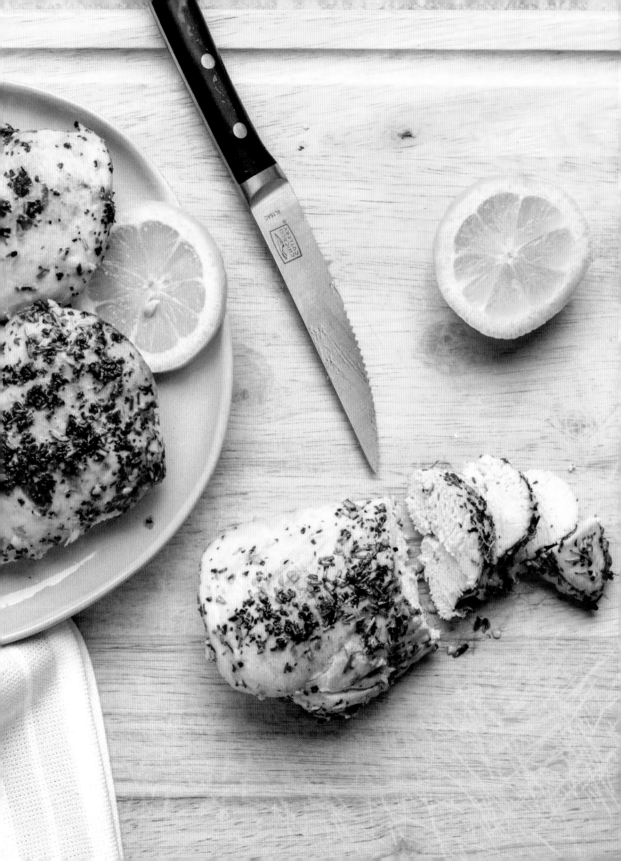

# BARBECUE CHICKEN WITH BAKED SWEET POTATOES AND STEAMED COLLARD GREENS

DF | GF | NF

MAKES 4 SERVINGS

3 tablespoons extra-virgin olive oil

Juice of ½ lemon

1 teaspoon minced garlic

1 tablespoon smoked paprika

1½ pounds boneless, skinless chicken breasts

⅓ cup barbecue sauce, such as The New Primal

Baked Sweet Potatoes (recipe follows), for serving

Steamed Collard Greens (recipe follows), for serving

In a small bowl, whisk together the oil, lemon juice, garlic, and paprika. Transfer to a large resealable plastic bag. Add the chicken, seal the bag, and transfer to the refrigerator to marinate for at least 1 hour or as long as overnight.

Preheat the oven to 350°F. Line a rimmed baking sheet with parchment paper or aluminum foil.

Transfer the chicken to the prepared baking sheet and bake for 20 minutes. Remove the baking sheet from the oven and use a basting brush or spatula to spread half of the barbecue sauce on the chicken. Bake for 5 minutes. Brush the remaining barbecue sauce on the chicken. Bake for 5 more minutes, or until the chicken is cooked through.

Serve the chicken with the sweet potatoes and collard greens.

COOKING TIP: The chicken and sweet potatoes can be baked at the same time, and you can make the collard greens while they're in the oven.

## BAKED SWEET POTATOES

DF | GF | NF | V

**MAKES 4 SERVINGS**

4 medium sweet potatoes, chopped

2 tablespoons avocado oil

¼ teaspoon garlic powder

¼ teaspoon smoked or sweet paprika

⅛ teaspoon sea salt

⅛ teaspoon black pepper

Preheat the oven to 350°F. Line a rimmed baking sheet with aluminum foil or parchment paper.

Put the potatoes in a large mixing bowl. Add the oil, garlic powder, paprika, salt, and pepper and toss to coat well.

Transfer the potatoes to the prepared baking sheet. Bake for 25 minutes, flip the potatoes, then bake for 15 minutes more, until golden brown. Serve.

## STEAMED COLLARD GREENS

DF | GF | NF | V | 30 | OP

**MAKES 4 SERVINGS**

1 bunch collard greens

1 teaspoon extra-virgin olive oil

½ teaspoon minced garlic

3 tablespoons water

2 teaspoons everything bagel seasoning

Cut along the center rib of each collard green leaf to remove the leaves. Discard the ribs. Stack the leaves and roll them up, then cut crosswise into small ribbons.

Heat the oil in a large skillet over medium-high heat. Add the garlic and cook for about 1 minute, until fragrant. Add the greens and water. Reduce the heat to medium-low, cover, and steam, stirring occasionally, for 3 to 5 minutes, until the greens are tender.

Serve the greens sprinkled with the seasoning.

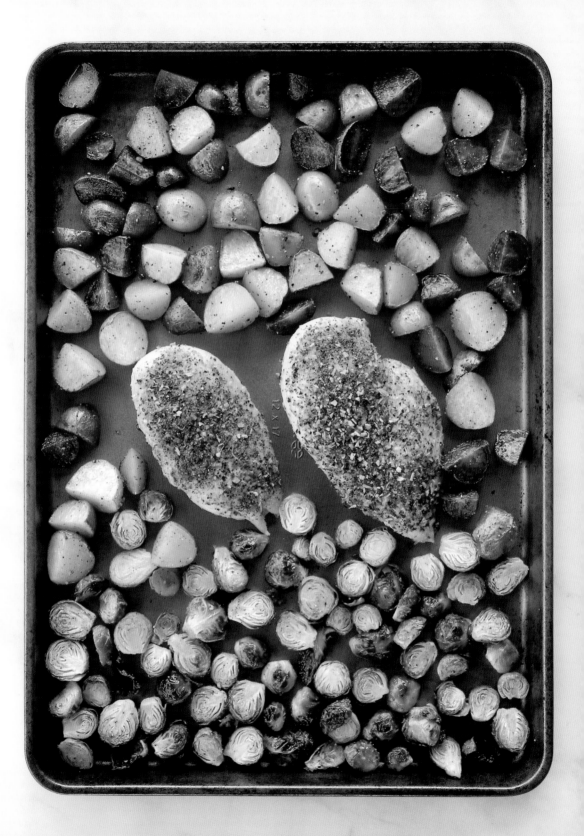

# ONE-PAN CHICKEN AND VEGGIE DINNER

DF | GF | NF

**1 pound boneless, skinless chicken breasts**

**2 tablespoons avocado oil or extra-virgin olive oil, divided**

**2 tablespoons Italian seasoning blend or Trader Joe's 21 Seasoning Salute**

**Sea salt and black pepper, to taste**

**2 pounds petite rainbow potatoes, halved**

**1 cup halved Brussels sprouts**

Preheat the oven to 400°F. Line a rimmed baking sheet with parchment paper or lightly spray with olive oil cooking spray.

Put the chicken breasts on the prepared baking sheet and drizzle with 1 tablespoon of the oil. Sprinkle with the seasoning blend, salt, and pepper.

In a large bowl, toss together the potatoes, the sprouts, the remaining 1 tablespoon of oil, and the salt and pepper. Scatter the vegetables on the baking sheet around the chicken.

Bake for 25 minutes, or until the potatoes are lightly browned and the chicken is cooked through. Serve.

---

**COOKING TIP:** To make this vegan, use a 15-ounce package of extra-firm tofu, drained and chopped, instead of the chicken. The cooking time will be closer to 30 to 35 minutes.

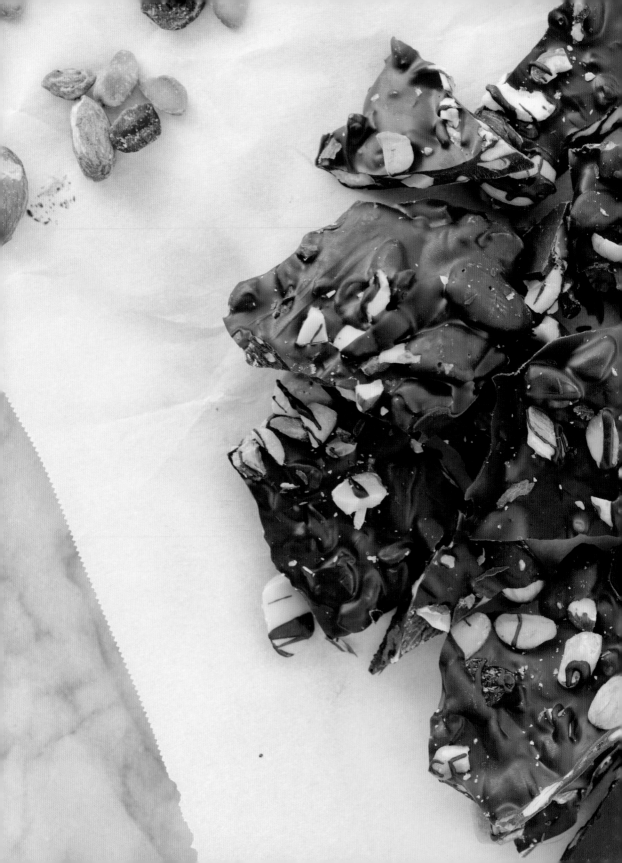

# CHAPTER NINE

# PERFORMANCE SNACKS AND SWEET TREATS

If you have a sweet tooth like me, this may quickly become your favorite chapter of the book. And the best part about all of these savory snacks and sweet treats is they're created with all wholesome ingredients. These snacks and desserts feature fresh fruit and even vegetables, like blueberries, banana, avocado, dates, and zucchini. The first few recipes in this chapter are great to have on hand pre- or post-workout. The post-workout recovery bites and homemade sports drinks are two favorites of my clients. If you're going to be cooking for a crowd, I recommend the cashew queso or a double batch of the no-bake brownies. Some of these sweet treats can also double as a breakfast, especially the almond zucchini muffins and chocolate chip banana bread.

# POST-WORKOUT RECOVERY BITES

**DF | GF | V | NK | OP**

**MAKES 20 BITES**

**2 cups old-fashioned rolled oats**

**1 ripe banana, mashed**

**½ cup creamy peanut butter**

**2 tablespoons honey (optional)**

**1 scoop plant-based or whey protein powder of choice**

**1 tablespoon chia seeds or ground flaxseed**

In a large bowl, combine all the ingredients and mix well. Cover and refrigerate for 1 hour, then use your hands to roll the mixture into 20 tablespoon-size balls. Store in an airtight container in the refrigerator for up to 1 week.

---

**NUTRITION TIP:** Be sure to choose NSF Certified for Sport or Informed Sport protein powders. Some examples include Klean Athlete, Momentous, Ladder, BiPro, NOW Sports, and Garden of Life Sport. If gluten is a concern, seek out oats that are certified gluten-free.

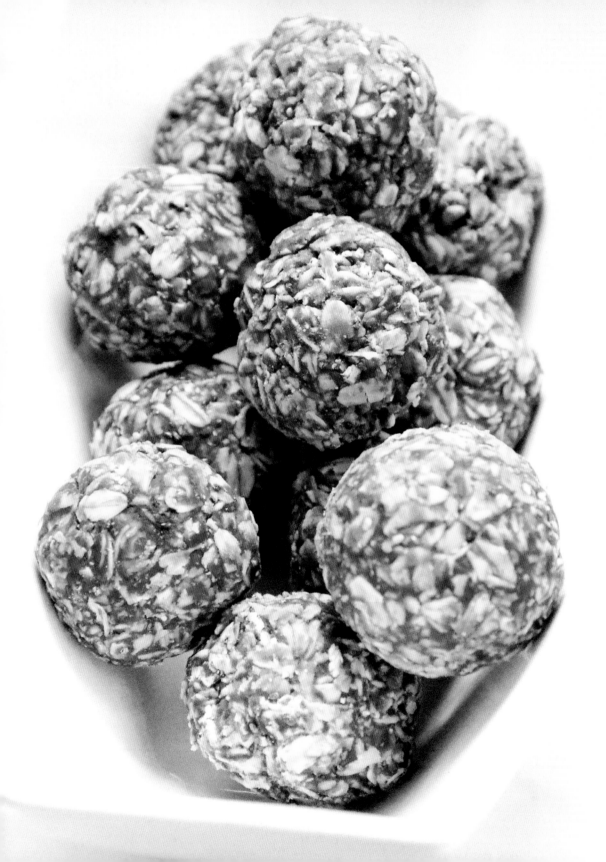

# HOMEMADE SPORTS DRINKS

**DF | GF | NF | V | 30 | NK | OP**

## CITRUS SPORTS DRINK

Juice of 4 oranges or
1 cup no-sugar-added
orange juice

Juice of ½ lemon

¾ cup coconut water

⅛ teaspoon salt

Stir together all the ingredients in a glass. Drink immediately, or refrigerate for up to 1 day. Stir again before drinking.

## WATERMELON SPORTS DRINK

1½ cups chopped
watermelon

1 cup coconut water

Juice of ½ lime

⅛ teaspoon salt

Combine all the ingredients in a blender. Blend until smooth, then enjoy immediately.

---

**PERFORMANCE TIP:** There is 2,325 mg sodium in 1 teaspoon salt. Using ⅛ teaspoon salt in these sports drinks provides roughly 290 mg sodium. Using ¼ teaspoon would provide roughly 580 mg sodium. Adjust if you need more or less, depending on your sweat rate and if you are a heavier sweater. To compare, 20 ounces of Gatorade provides about 270 mg sodium.

# 3-INGREDIENT ENERGY BARS

**DF | GF | V | NK**

MAKES 12 BARS (2 BARS PER SERVING)

½ cup pitted Medjool dates

¼ cup raw almonds

3 tablespoons creamy peanut butter

Line a baking dish with parchment paper cut so that two sides have a bit of overhang. You'll use these as handles later. Choose the size of the dish based on how thick or thin you'd like the bars.

Put the dates in a food processor and process until they form a thick paste. Add the almonds and peanut butter and process until well combined.

Press the mixture into the prepared dish, using your fingers or the back of a spoon to smooth it out evenly. Cover and refrigerate for 30 minutes. Cut into 12 bars when ready to eat. Alternatively, to make balls, use your hands to roll the mixture into tablespoon-size balls.

Store in an airtight container in the refrigerator for up to 1 week or in the freezer for up to 3 months.

---

**COOKING TIP:** You can buy Medjool dates that are already pitted to save time.

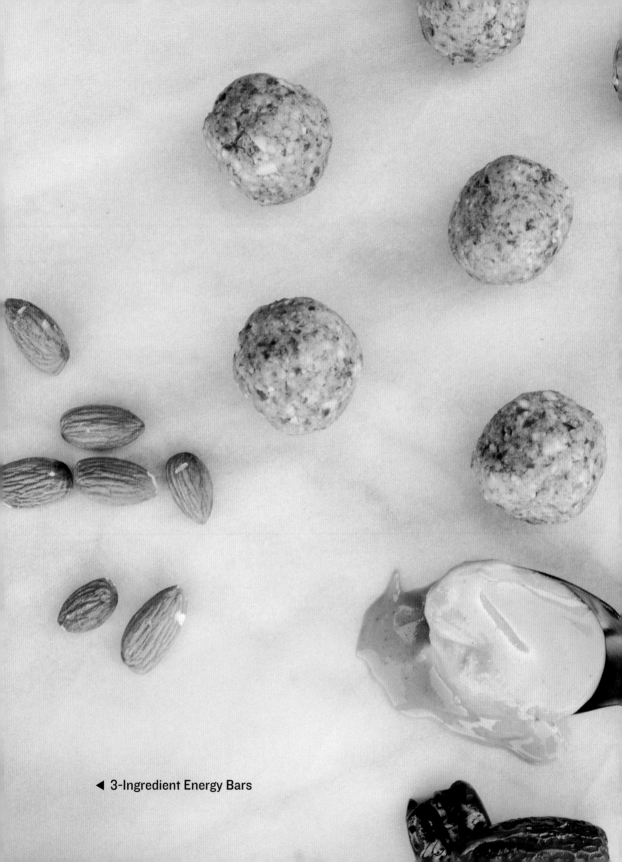

◀ 3-Ingredient Energy Bars

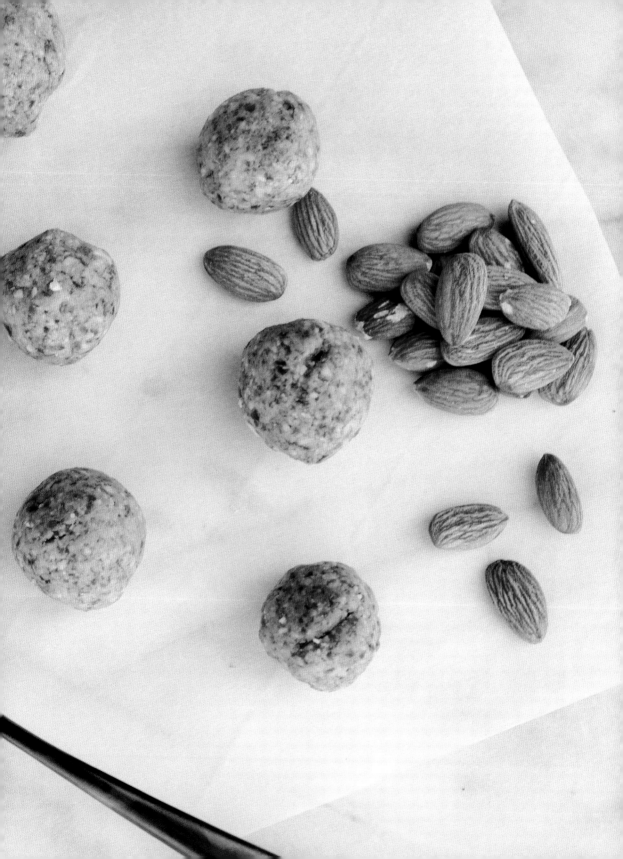

# ENDURANCE TRAIL MIX

DF | GF | V | 30 | NK | OP

MAKES 10 (½-CUP) SERVINGS

2 cups breakfast cereal of choice
(gluten-free if necessary)

1 cup almonds

1 cup cashews

½ cup peanuts or pistachios

½ cup pumpkin seeds or sunflower
seeds

Combine all the ingredients in a
large airtight container and toss to
mix. If desired, transfer to individual
grab-and-go bags or containers. Store
at room temperature for up to 1 month.

# PARMESAN-ROASTED EDAMAME

GF | NF | VEG

MAKES 4 SERVINGS

1 (10-ounce) package fresh or thawed
frozen shelled edamame

1 tablespoon extra-virgin olive oil

¼ cup grated parmesan cheese

¼ teaspoon garlic powder

¼ teaspoon black pepper

Pinch of sea salt (optional)

Preheat the oven to 400°F. Line a
rimmed baking sheet with parchment paper.

In a large bowl, toss the edamame
with the oil, parmesan, pepper, garlic
powder, and salt (if using) until
evenly coated.

Spread out the edamame in a single
layer on the prepared baking sheet.
Roast for 15 minutes, then shake the
pan and roast for an additional 10 to
15 minutes, until the edamame are
crispy. Allow to cool.

Store in an airtight container in the
refrigerator for up to 5 days.

COOKING TIP: For a spicy kick, swap out the
garlic powder for ¼ teaspoon of chili powder
or red pepper flakes.

# ROASTED CHICKPEAS

**DF | GF | NF | V**

2 (15-ounce) cans chickpeas, rinsed, drained, and patted dry

2 tablespoons avocado oil

¼ teaspoon onion powder

¼ teaspoon garlic powder

¼ teaspoon smoked paprika

¼ teaspoon ground cumin

⅛ teaspoon sea salt

Preheat the oven to 400°F. Line a rimmed baking sheet with parchment paper.

In a large bowl, toss the chickpeas with the oil, onion powder, garlic powder, paprika, cumin, and salt and mix until evenly coated.

Spread out the chickpeas in a single layer on the prepared baking sheet and roast for 10 minutes. Shake the pan, then roast for another 15 minutes, or until the chickpeas are crispy. Allow to cool.

Store in an airtight container at room temperature for up to 5 days.

# CASHEW QUESO

DF | GF | V | 30

1 cup raw cashews

½ cup nutritional yeast

1–2 cups water, divided

Juice of ½ lemon

1 tomato, finely chopped

¼ cup chopped fresh cilantro

1 tablespoon garlic powder

1 tablespoon onion powder

1 tablespoon smoked or sweet paprika

1 teaspoon cayenne pepper

½ teaspoon sea salt

½ teaspoon black pepper

Plantain or tortilla chips, for serving

Put the cashews in a small saucepan and cover with water. Bring to a boil over high heat and cook for 8 minutes. Drain, then transfer the cashews to a high-speed blender or food processor. Add the nutritional yeast and 1 cup fresh water. Puree until smooth.

Pour the cashew mixture into the same saucepan and add the lemon juice, tomato, cilantro, garlic powder, onion powder, paprika, cayenne, salt, and black pepper. Stir well and heat over medium-low heat, adding as much of the remaining 1 cup of water as needed to reach your desired consistency.

Serve warm with plantain chips or tortilla chips.

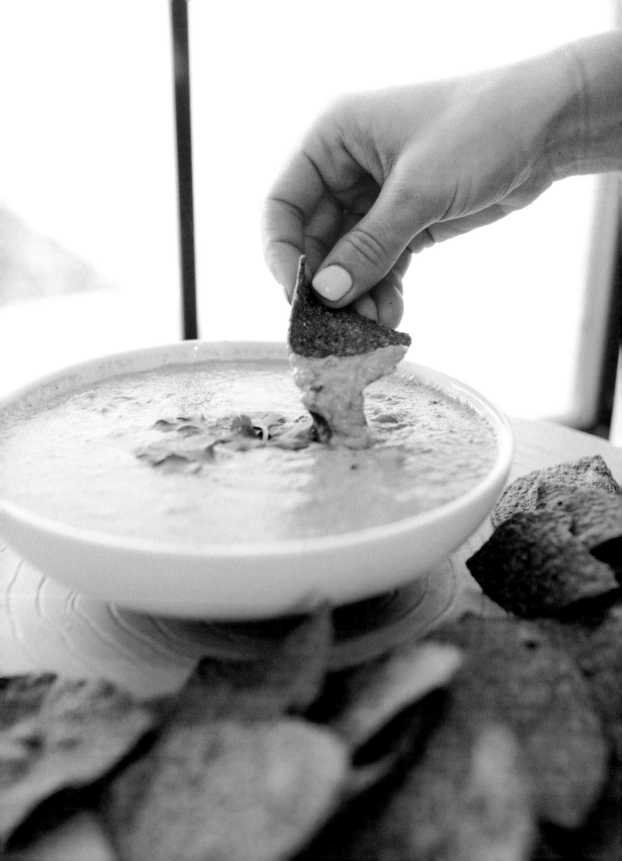

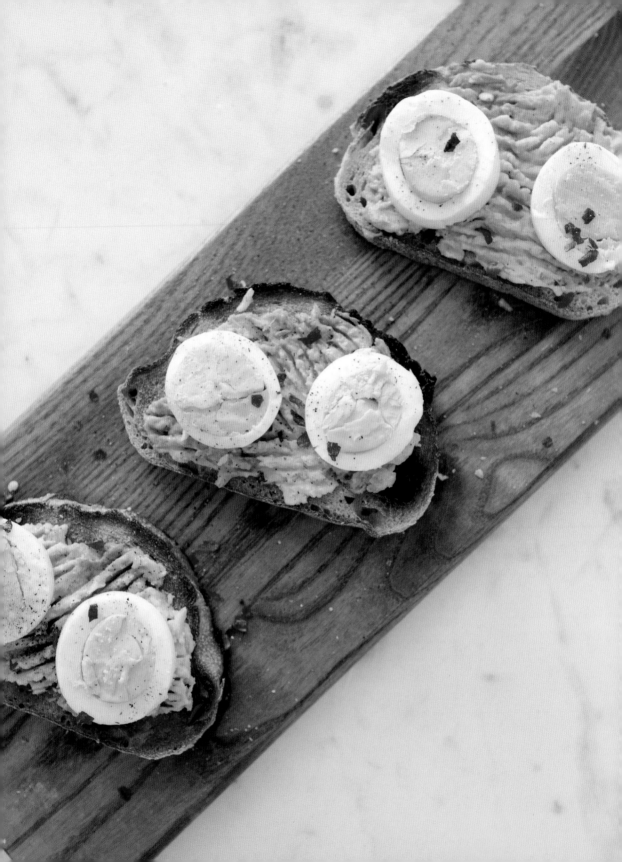

# AVOCADO TOAST WITH HARD-BOILED EGGS

**DF | NF | VEG | 30**

4 large eggs

2 slices sprouted grain bread, such as Ezekiel

1 small avocado, pitted and peeled

½ teaspoon red pepper flakes

¼ teaspoon sea salt

¼ teaspoon black pepper

Put the eggs in a saucepan and cover with water. Bring to a boil over high heat. Immediately remove the pan from the heat, cover, and let stand for 12 minutes. Use a slotted spoon to transfer the eggs to a bowl of ice water. Peel the eggs and slice into rounds.

Meanwhile, toast the bread.

Using a fork, mash half of the avocado on each slice of toast. Top each with the hard-boiled egg slices, then sprinkle on the red pepper flakes, salt, and black pepper.

---

**COOKING TIP:** Hard-boiled eggs can be stored for up to 1 week in your refrigerator. To keep leftover avocado from browning in your refrigerator, sprinkle with fresh lemon or lime juice and store in an airtight container.

# ALMOND ZUCCHINI MUFFINS

**DF | GF | VEG**

1¾ cups almond flour

1½ teaspoons baking soda

1½ teaspoons ground cinnamon

½ teaspoon ground nutmeg

½ teaspoon sea salt

1 banana, mashed

3 large eggs, at room temperature

3 tablespoons honey

1 tablespoon melted coconut oil

1 cup grated zucchini

Preheat the oven to 350°F. Line a 12-cup standard muffin tin with parchment or silicone cupcake liners.

In a large bowl, whisk together the almond flour, baking soda, cinnamon, nutmeg, and salt.

In a separate bowl, combine the banana, eggs, honey, and oil. Using a handheld electric mixer, beat on medium speed until smooth, 2 to 3 minutes. Whisk in the flour mixture until just combined.

Pat the grated zucchini with paper towels to remove as much moisture as possible. Add the zucchini to the batter and fold it in until well combined.

Spoon the batter into the prepared muffin tin, filling each cup about three-quarters full. Bake for 20 to 25 minutes, until a toothpick inserted into the center of the muffins comes out clean. Transfer the muffins to a wire rack to cool for 5 to 10 minutes.

Store the muffins in an airtight container in the refrigerator for up to 1 week.

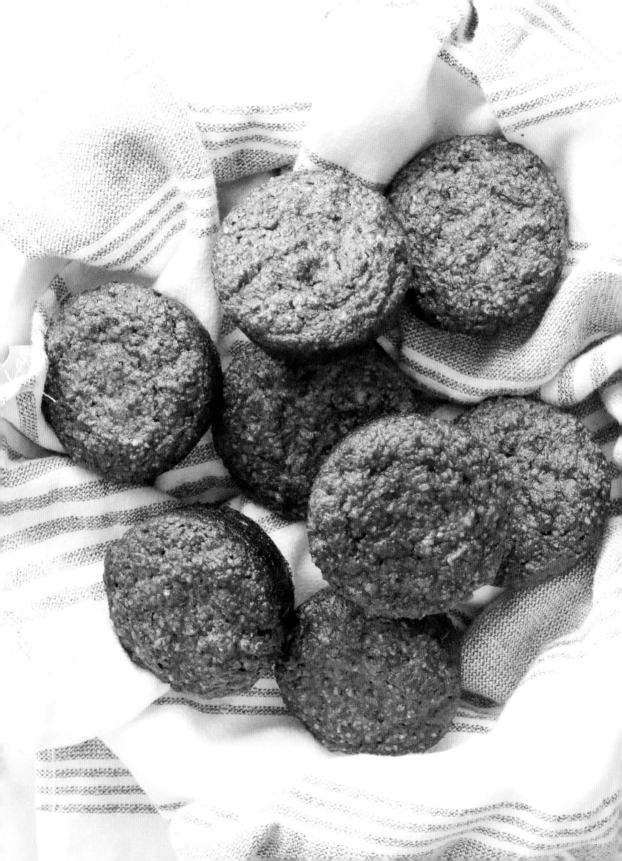

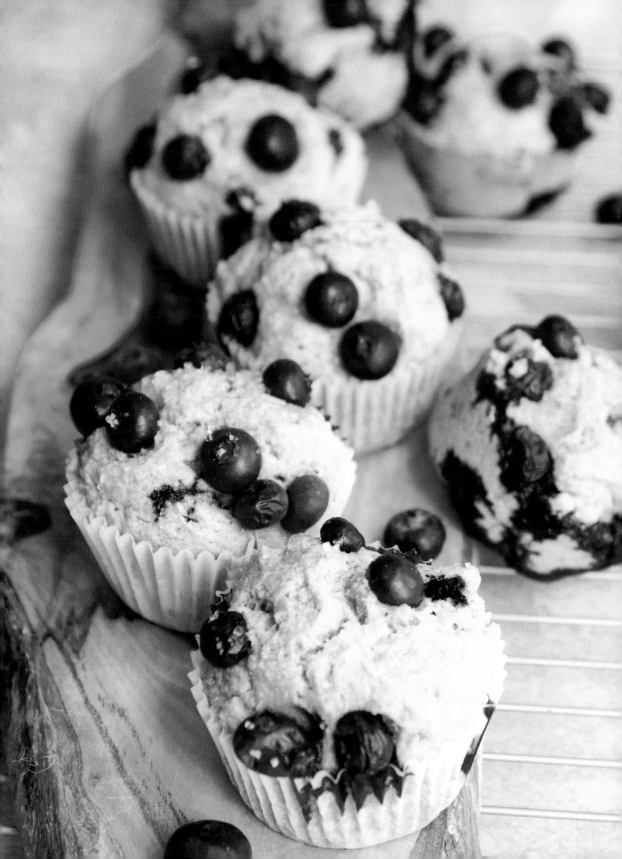

# BLUEBERRY MUFFINS

**DF | VEG**

⅔ cup unsweetened vanilla nondairy milk or 2% milk

1 large egg, at room temperature

⅓ cup avocado oil or melted coconut oil

⅓ cup pure maple syrup or honey

1 teaspoon apple cider vinegar

½ teaspoon vanilla extract

2 cups whole-wheat flour, gluten-free all-purpose flour, or oat flour

½ teaspoon baking powder

½ teaspoon baking soda

¼ teaspoon sea salt

1 heaping cup fresh or frozen blueberries

Coconut sugar, for sprinkling (optional)

Preheat the oven to 375°F. Line a 12-cup standard muffin tin with parchment or silicone cupcake liners.

In a large bowl, whisk together the milk, egg, oil, maple syrup, vinegar, and vanilla.

In a separate bowl, whisk together the flour, baking powder, baking soda, and salt. Use a large spoon or spatula to stir the flour mixture into the milk mixture until just combined. Do not overmix. Fold in the blueberries, keeping a few aside to place on top.

Spoon the batter into the prepared muffin tin, filling each cup about three-quarters full. Top with the reserved blueberries and a sprinkle of coconut sugar (if using).

Bake for 19 to 22 minutes, until a toothpick inserted into the center of the muffins comes out clean. Allow to cool in the tin for a few minutes, then transfer to a wire rack to cool completely.

Store the muffins in an airtight container in the refrigerator for up to 1 week.

---

**COOKING TIP:** If you prefer your muffins to be very moist, add a mashed small ripe banana to the milk mixture before adding the dry ingredients.

# CHOCOLATE CHIP BANANA BREAD

**DF | GF | VEG**

**4 ripe bananas**

**2 large eggs, at room temperature**

**¼ cup creamy almond butter**

**2 tablespoons pure maple syrup or honey**

**2 cups almond flour**

**2 teaspoons baking powder**

**¼ teaspoon sea salt**

**½ cup dairy-free dark chocolate chips, such as Enjoy Life**

Preheat the oven to 350°F. Lightly coat a 9-inch loaf pan with olive oil cooking spray.

Mash the bananas in a large bowl. Add the eggs, almond butter, and maple syrup and mix well.

In a separate bowl, combine the almond flour, baking powder, and salt. Whisk the flour mixture into the egg mixture until just combined. Fold in the chocolate chips, keeping a few aside to place on top.

Pour the batter into the prepared loaf pan and add the reserved chocolate chips on top. Bake for 35 minutes. Let cool completely before cutting into 12 slices.

Store in an airtight container in the refrigerator for up to 1 week.

---

**COOKING TIP:** If you do not have a loaf pan, you can use the same batter to make muffins. Line a 12-cup standard muffin tin with parchment or silicone cupcake liners and reduce the baking time to 20 to 22 minutes.

# ALMOND FLOUR CHOCOLATE CHIP COOKIES

**DF | GF | VEG | 30**

**2 cups almond flour (or 1 cup almond flour and 1 cup old-fashioned rolled oats)**

**½ teaspoon baking soda**

**¼ teaspoon sea salt**

**1 large egg, at room temperature**

**⅓ cup pure maple syrup**

**2 tablespoons melted coconut oil**

**½ cup dairy-free dark chocolate chips, such as Enjoy Life**

Preheat the oven to 350°F. Line a rimmed baking sheet with parchment paper.

In a large bowl, whisk together the almond flour, baking soda, and salt. In a separate bowl, whisk together the egg, maple syrup, and oil.

Whisk the flour mixture into the egg mixture until well combined. Fold in the chocolate chips.

Using a tablespoon, portion out the dough into 12 cookies on the prepared baking sheet, leaving space between the cookies. Gently press down on each cookie to flatten.

Bake for 12 minutes, or until the edges have turned golden brown. Allow the cookies to cool for a few minutes on the baking sheet before transferring to a wire rack to cool completely.

Store in an airtight container at room temperature for up to 3 days or in the refrigerator for up to 1 week.

# RAW COOKIE DOUGH

**DF | GF | V | 30 | NK**

½ cup raw cashews

2 tablespoons old-fashioned rolled oats or oat flour

3 tablespoons creamy almond butter

2 tablespoons pure maple syrup

2–3 tablespoons water

2 teaspoons vanilla extract

⅛ teaspoon baking soda

⅛ teaspoon sea salt

3 tablespoons dairy-free dark chocolate chips, such as Enjoy Life

Soak the cashews in warm water for 30 minutes. Drain and pat dry with paper towels.

Transfer the cashews to a food processor. Add the oats, the almond butter, the maple syrup, 2 tablespoons of water, the vanilla, the baking soda, and the salt and pulse until the consistency resembles cookie dough. Add up to 1 tablespoon of additional water as needed.

Stir in the chocolate chips with a large spoon.

Store in an airtight container in the refrigerator for up to 1 week or in the freezer for up to 2 months.

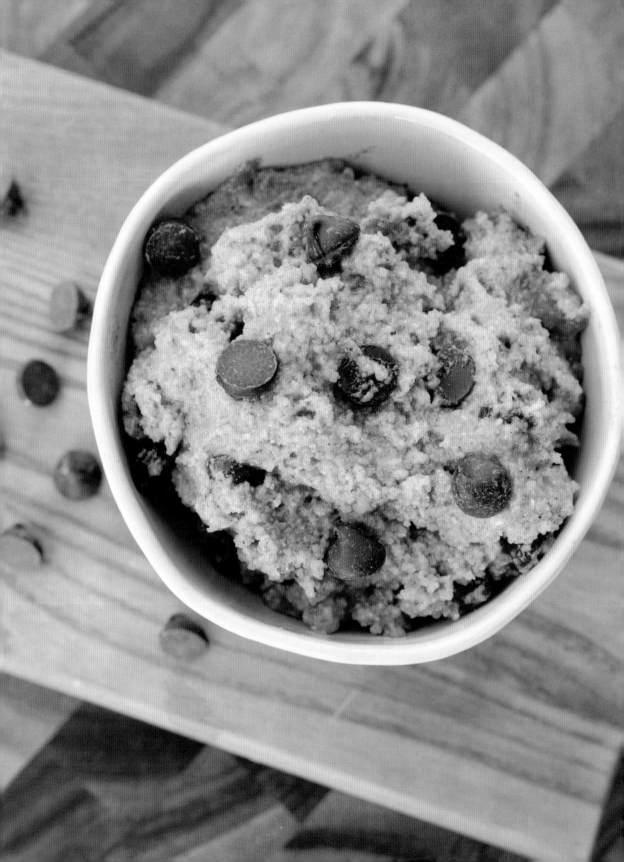

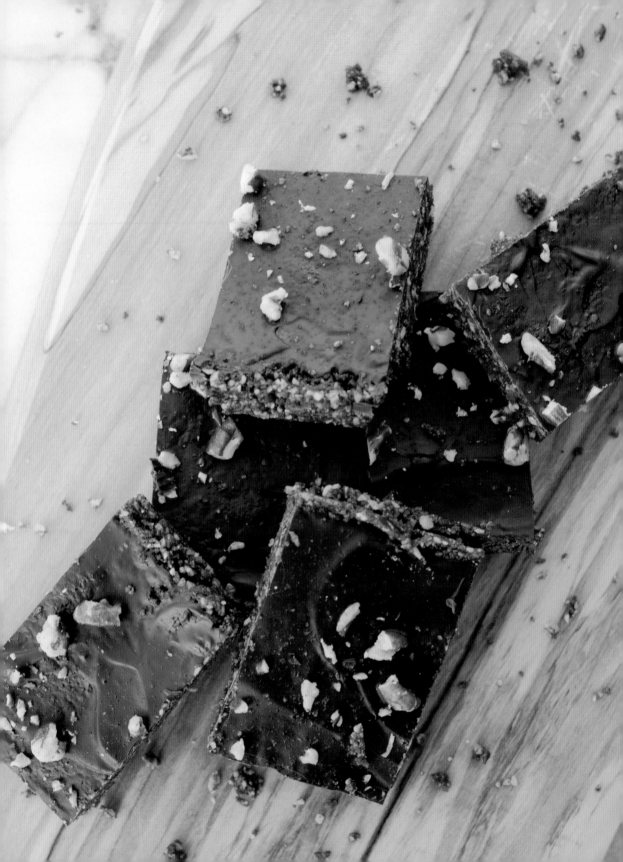

# NO-BAKE BROWNIES

DF | GF | V | 30 | NK

1¼ cups chopped walnuts, plus more for topping

¼ cup almonds

1½ cups pitted Medjool dates

⅓ cup raw cacao powder

½ teaspoon vanilla extract

1 (1.5-ounce) dairy-free dark chocolate bar

⅛ teaspoon coarse salt

Line an 8-inch square baking pan with parchment paper or aluminum foil, allowing it to hang over the edges.

Combine the walnuts and almonds in a food processor and process until finely ground but not so much that it turns into a paste.

Add the dates, cacao powder, and vanilla and process until well combined. The texture will be crumbly. Transfer the mixture to the prepared baking pan and spread evenly, firmly pressing down to make an even layer.

Put the chocolate in a glass bowl and melt on medium power in the microwave for 90 seconds. Stir and add more time as needed in 30-second increments until the chocolate has completely melted.

Drizzle the melted chocolate on top of the brownie mixture and use a spatula to spread it out evenly. Top with the salt and a few more chopped walnuts.

Cover and refrigerate for a few hours before cutting and serving. Store in the refrigerator for up to 1 week.

# VEGAN PEANUT BUTTER COOKIES

**DF | GF | V | 30**

**1 tablespoon ground flaxseed**

**3 tablespoons water**

**¾ cup pitted Medjool dates**

**¾ cup creamy peanut butter**

**½ cup chopped walnuts**

**1 teaspoon vanilla extract**

**½ teaspoon baking soda**

**¼ teaspoon baking powder**

**Sea salt, for sprinkling**

Preheat the oven to 350°F. Line a rimmed baking sheet with parchment paper.

To make the "flax egg," in a small bowl, gently whisk together the flaxseed and water and refrigerate for 10 to 15 minutes.

In a food processor, pulse the dates to make a paste. Add the flax egg, peanut butter, walnuts, vanilla, baking soda, and baking powder and pulse until just combined. Do not overprocess.

Use a tablespoon to scoop the dough into your hands. Roll into balls, then press them flat onto the prepared baking sheet. You should get about 12 cookies.

Bake for 12 to 14 minutes, until the edges are just golden brown. While the cookies are still hot, sprinkle a bit of salt on top and let cool for at least 5 minutes.

Store in an airtight container at room temperature for up to 3 days or in the refrigerator for up to 1 week.

---

**COOKING TIP:** Flax eggs are a vegan alternative to chicken eggs. If you prefer to use a chicken egg in this recipe, that will work well here, too.

# SLOW COOKER PEACH-APPLE CRISP

**DF | GF | VEG | NK**

3 large peaches, pitted and chopped

3 large apples, cored and chopped

1 teaspoon plus 3 tablespoons honey, divided

1½ teaspoons ground cinnamon, divided

1¼ cups old-fashioned rolled oats

¼ cup almond flour

3 tablespoons melted coconut oil

½ teaspoon vanilla extract

Dairy-free ice cream or frozen yogurt, for serving (optional)

In a large bowl, toss the peaches and apples with 1 teaspoon of the honey and 1 teaspoon of the cinnamon.

Lightly coat the bottom of a slow cooker with oil. Pour in the apple-peach mixture, spreading it out evenly.

In a large bowl, mix together the oats, the almond flour, the oil, the vanilla, the remaining 3 tablespoons of honey, and the remaining ½ teaspoon of cinnamon. The texture will be crumbly. Scatter the mixture evenly on top of the apple-peach mixture.

Place a paper towel between the slow cooker and the lid to help collect condensation. Cover and cook on high for 2 hours, or until the oats have turned golden brown.

Serve warm with ice cream on top, if you like.

---

**COOKING TIP:** This dessert can also be made in the oven. Assemble the crisp in a greased 8-inch baking dish and bake at 350°F for 35 to 45 minutes.

# DARK CHOCOLATE NUT CLUSTERS

**DF | GF | V | NK**

**2 (1.5-ounce) dairy-free dark chocolate bars**

**¼ cup pistachios, finely chopped or crushed**

**¼ cup cashews, finely chopped or crushed**

**¼ cup almonds, finely chopped or crushed**

**2 tablespoons dried cranberries**

**¼ cup other nuts of choice, such as walnuts or macadamia nuts, finely chopped or crushed (optional)**

Line a rimmed baking sheet with parchment paper.

Break the chocolate into pieces and put them in a glass bowl. Melt on medium power in the microwave for 90 seconds. Stir and add more time as needed in 30-second increments until the chocolate has completely melted.

Add the nuts and cranberries to the bowl of melted chocolate and stir to coat. Pour the mixture onto the prepared baking sheet and spread using a flat spatula until it is about ½ inch thick. Scrape out the bowl, reserving 1 tablespoon of melted chocolate to drizzle on top.

Scatter a few additional nuts (if using) on top, then drizzle with the reserved chocolate. Refrigerate for 30 to 60 minutes, until completely hardened. Break apart into small pieces.

Store in an airtight container at cool room temperature or in the refrigerator for up to 1 month.

---

**NUTRITION TIP:** Dark chocolate is rich in magnesium and flavonoids. Flavonoids are a large group of antioxidants, and the ones specifically found in cocoa beans are called flavanols. Choose 70 percent or higher dark chocolate for the highest flavanol content.

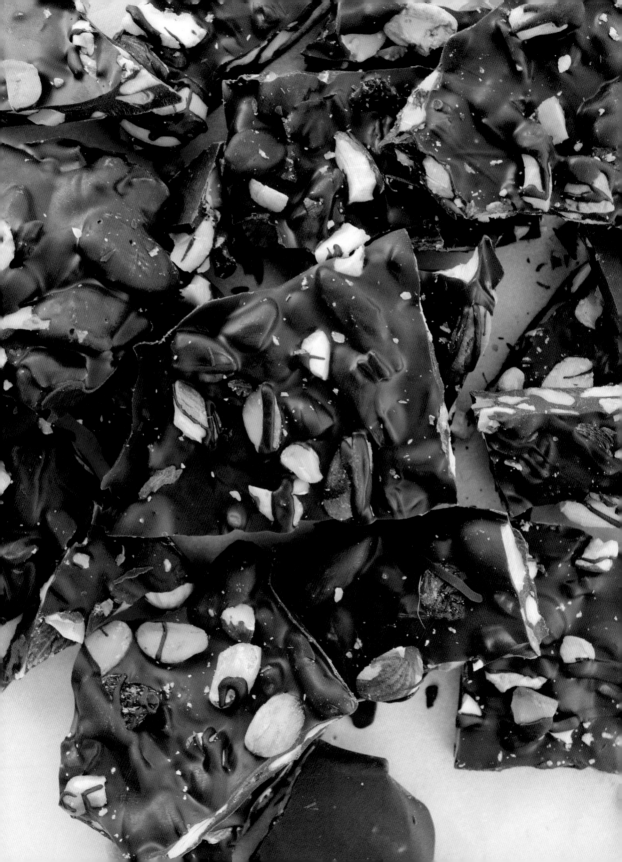

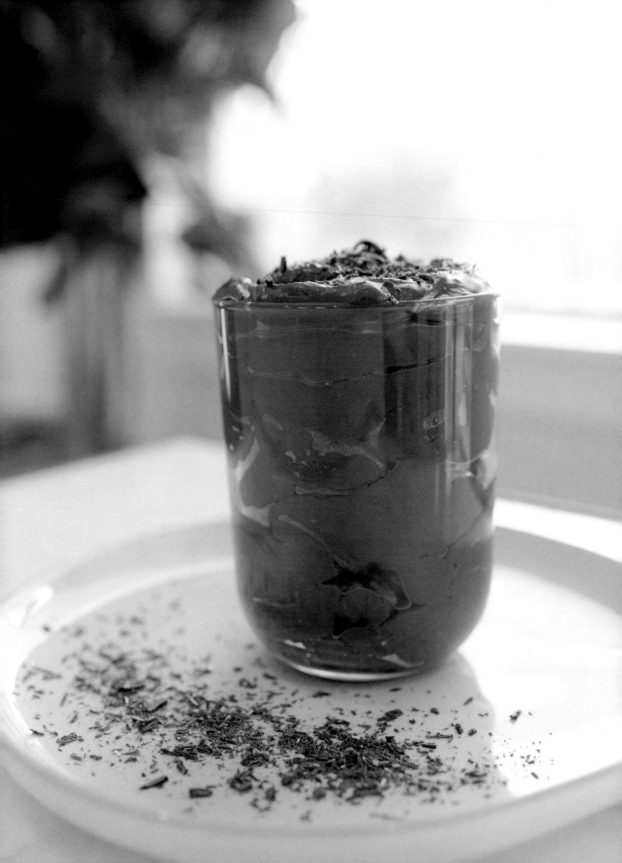

# AVOCADO MOUSSE

**DF | GF | V | NK**

½ cup dairy-free dark chocolate chips, such as Enjoy Life

2 small ripe avocados, pitted and peeled

3 tablespoons cacao powder or unsweetened cocoa powder

⅓ cup unsweetened nondairy milk or 2% milk

¼ cup pure maple syrup

2 tablespoons creamy peanut butter (optional)

1 teaspoon vanilla extract

Raspberries, pomegranate seeds, or dark chocolate shavings, for topping (optional)

Put the chocolate chips in a glass bowl and melt on medium power in the microwave for 90 seconds. Stir and add more time as needed in 30-second increments until the chocolate has completely melted. Set aside to cool slightly.

Transfer the chocolate to a food processor or blender and add the avocados, cacao powder, milk, maple syrup, peanut butter (if using), and vanilla. Puree until very smooth.

Taste and add more maple syrup if you prefer it sweeter, or add a little more milk for a thinner, smoother mousse.

Transfer the mixture to a bowl, cover, and refrigerate for at least 1 hour. To serve, spoon into a small dish and top with raspberries (if using).

Store in an airtight container in the refrigerator for up to 3 days or in the freezer for up to 3 weeks.

# FROZEN BERRY YOGURT BITES

**GF | NF | VEG | OP**

MAKES 6 (½-CUP) SERVINGS

**3 cups fresh blueberries**

**½ cup plain Greek yogurt or dairy-free yogurt**

Line a rimmed baking sheet with parchment paper.

Pierce the center of a blueberry with a toothpick, then dip it into the yogurt until fully coated. Slide the blueberry off the toothpick and onto the parchment paper. Repeat with the rest of the blueberries.

Freeze for at least 1 hour, until hardened.

Store in an airtight container in the freezer for up to 1 month.

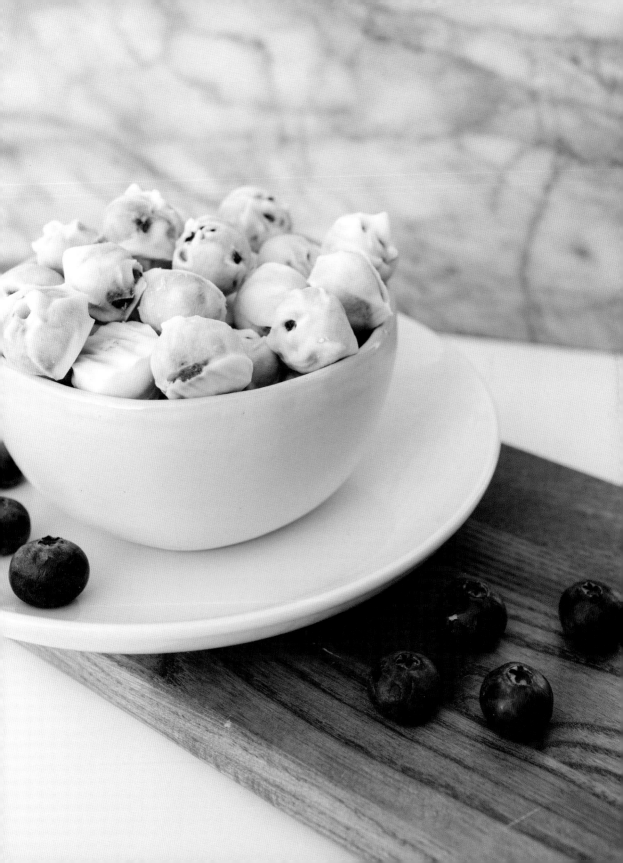

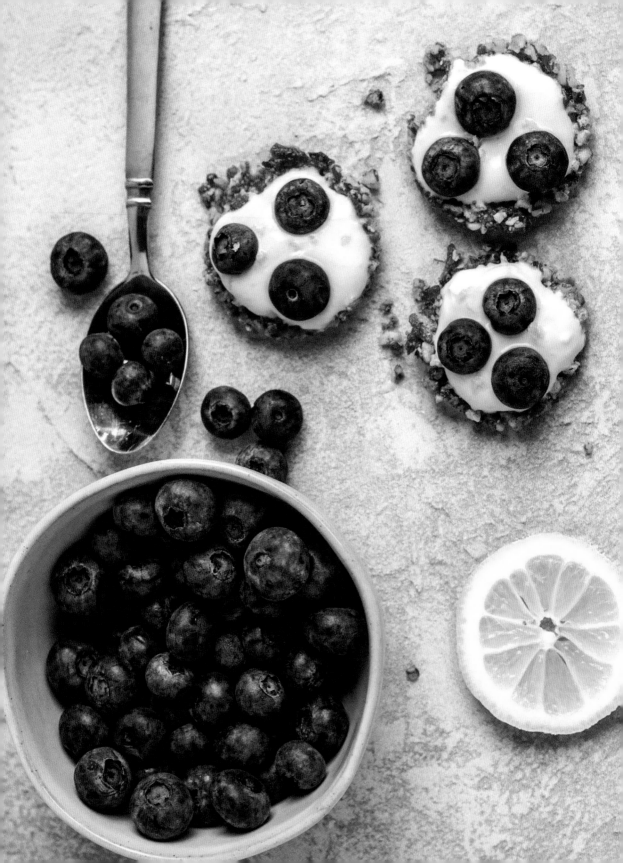

# BLUEBERRY-LEMON TARTS

**GF | VEG**

MAKES 12 TARTS

1 cup pecans

½ cup cashews

½ cup pitted Medjool dates

½ teaspoon ground cinnamon

Pinch of sea salt

1 cup plain Greek yogurt or dairy-free yogurt

1½ tablespoons honey

½ teaspoon vanilla extract

½ teaspoon grated lemon zest

1 teaspoon freshly squeezed lemon juice

1 cup fresh blueberries

Line a 12-cup standard muffin tin with parchment or silicone cupcake liners.

In a food processor, pulse the pecans, cashews, dates, cinnamon, and salt until crumbly. Press the mixture firmly into the bottom of each cupcake liner. Freeze for at least 1 hour and preferably overnight. (The firmer the better, as the crust softens quickly.)

Meanwhile, in a bowl, whisk together the yogurt, honey, vanilla, lemon zest, and lemon juice. Cover and refrigerate until ready to use.

Gently remove the liners from the muffin tin and transfer them to a plate. Scoop a small spoonful of the yogurt filling on top of the crust in each cup. Top each with a few blueberries.

Store in the freezer for up to 1 week. Allow to thaw for a few minutes before enjoying.

# RECIPE NUTRITIONAL INFORMATION

*Nutrient analysis for each recipe was performed using the ESHA food processor database. Variations may occur due to food preparation, substitutions, and brand or type of ingredients used. All calculations are shown for single servings. Calculations for entrées are also shown for weight gain servings (twice the amount of food in a single serving). All recipes that call for any type of milk were made with unsweetened almond milk.*

## CHAPTER 5: THE PERFECT SMOOTHIE

**Simple Green Smoothie made with 1 scoop whey protein**

| | |
|---|---|
| Calories | 264 kcal |
| Carbs | 21 g |
| Protein | 21 g |
| Fat | 11 g |
| Sodium | 230 mg |
| Fiber | 7 g |
| Calcium | 617 mg |
| Vitamin C | 41 mg |
| Vitamin A | 3764 IU |
| Vitamin E | 16 IU |
| Vitamin K | 227.72 mcg |
| Vitamin B12 | 3 mcg |

**Berry-Beet Smoothie made with 1 scoop whey protein**

| | |
|---|---|
| Calories | 301 kcal |
| Carbs | 45 g |
| Protein | 25 g |
| Fat | 4 g |
| Sodium | 290 mg |
| Fiber | 6 g |
| Vitamin C | 50 mg |
| Calcium | 595 mg |
| Vitamin E | 16 IU |
| Vitamin B12 | 3 mcg |

**Gut Health Berry Smoothie made with unsweetened almond milk and 1 scoop vanilla plant-based protein powder**

| | |
|---|---|
| Calories | 373 kcal |
| Carbs | 45 g |
| Protein | 28 g |
| Fat | 13 g |
| Sodium | 359 mg |
| Fiber | 12 g |
| Vitamin C | 48 mg |
| Calcium | 929 mg |
| Vitamin B12 | 5 mcg |

**Tropical Green Smoothie made with coconut water and 1 scoop whey protein**

| | |
|---|---|
| Calories | 411 kcal |
| Carbs | 52 g |
| Protein | 27 g |
| Fat | 14 g |
| Sodium | 160 g |
| Fiber | 11 g |
| Vitamin A | 6000 IU |
| Vitamin C | 102 mg |
| Vitamin K | 272 mcg |

**Citrus Antioxidant Smoothie**

| | |
|---|---|
| Calories | 260 kcal |
| Carbs | 68 g |
| Protein | 3 g |
| Fat | 0 g |
| Sodium | 110 mg |
| Fiber | 12 g |
| Vitamin A | 6767 IU |
| Vitamin C | 166 mg |
| Vitamin K | 272 mcg |

**Chocolate-Banana Smoothie made with 1 scoop whey protein**

| | |
|---|---|
| Calories | 460 kcal |
| Carbs | 37 g |
| Protein | 32 g |
| Fat | 21 g |
| Sodium | 370 mg |
| Fiber | 7 g |
| Vitamin A | 5898 IU |
| Vitamin C | 25 mg |
| Calcium | 627 mg |
| Vitamin E | 15 IU |
| Vitamin B12 | 3 mcg |
| Vitamin K | 273 mcg |

**Chocolate-Banana Smoothie made with 1 scoop whey protein and ½ cup oats**

| | |
|---|---|
| Calories | 610 kcal |
| Carbs | 64 g |
| Protein | 37 g |
| Fat | 24 g |
| Sodium | 370 mg |
| Fiber | 11 g |
| Vitamin A | 5898 IU |
| Vitamin C | 25 mg |
| Calcium | 647 mg |
| Vitamin E | 15 IU |
| Vitamin B12 | 3 mcg |
| Vitamin K | 273 mcg |

**Peppermint-Cacao Green Smoothie**

| | |
|---|---|
| Calories | 230 kcal |
| Carbs | 25 g |
| Protein | 7 g |
| Fat | 12 g |
| Sodium | 220 mg |
| Fiber | 6 g |
| Vitamin A | 5833 IU |
| Vitamin C | 23 mg |
| Calcium | 548 mg |
| Vitamin E | 12 IU |
| Vitamin B12 | 3 mcg |
| Vitamin K | 272 mcg |

**Coffee and Cacao Smoothie**

| | |
|---|---|
| Calories | 380 kcal |
| Carbs | 68 g |
| Protein | 9 g |
| Fat | 12 g |
| Sodium | 170 mg |
| Fiber | 6 g |
| Calcium | 535 mg |
| Vitamin E | 15 IU |
| Vitamin B12 | 3 mcg |

## CHAPTER 6: BREAKFAST

**Basic Overnight Oats**

| | |
|---|---|
| Calories | 390 kcal |
| Carbs | 57 g |
| Protein | 12 g |
| Fat | 16 g |
| Sodium | 110 mg |
| Fiber | 12 g |
| Calcium | 337 mg |
| Vitamin E | 14 IU |

**Morning Muesli**

| | |
|---|---|
| Calories | 520 kcal |
| Carbs | 76 g |
| Protein | 15 g |
| Fat | 19 g |
| Sodium | 180 mg |
| Fiber | 11 g |
| Calcium | 524 mg |
| Vitamin E | 29 IU |
| Vitamin B12 | 3 mcg |

*For Weight Gain*

| | |
|---|---|
| Calories | 1040 kcal |
| Carbs | 152 g |
| Protein | 30 g |
| Fat | 38 g |
| Sodium | 360 mg |
| Fiber | 22 g |
| Calcium | 1048 mg |
| Vitamin E | 58 IU |
| Vitamin B12 | 6 mcg |

**Sweet Potato and Black Bean Hash**

| | |
|---|---|
| Calories | 220 kcal |
| Carbs | 33 g |
| Protein | 7 g |
| Fat | 8 g |
| Sodium | 390 mg |
| Fiber | 8 g |

| Vitamin A | 9975 IU |
|---|---|
| Vitamin K | 37 mcg |

*For Weight Gain*

| Calories | 440 kcal |
|---|---|
| Carbs | 66 g |
| Protein | 14 g |
| Fat | 16 g |
| Sodium | 780 mg |
| Fiber | 16 g |
| Vitamin A | 19,950 IU |
| Vitamin K | 74 mcg |

**Farmers' Market Egg Casserole**

| Calories | 360 kcal |
|---|---|
| Carbs | 23 g |
| Protein | 11 g |
| Fat | 23 g |
| Sodium | 510 mg |
| Fiber | 3 g |
| Vitamin E | 13 IU |
| Vitamin B12 | 2 mcg |

*For Weight Gain*

| Calories | 720 kcal |
|---|---|
| Carbs | 46 g |
| Protein | 22 g |
| Fat | 46 g |
| Sodium | 1020 mg |
| Fiber | 6 g |
| Vitamin E | 26 IU |
| Vitamin B12 | 4 mcg |

**Breakfast Parfait made with 1 cup strawberries**

| Calories | 240 kcal |
|---|---|
| Carbs | 30 g |
| Protein | 18 g |
| Fat | 6 g |
| Sodium | 55 mg |
| Fiber | 5 g |
| Vitamin C | 98 mg |

**Baked Oatmeal Casserole**

| Calories | 410 kcal |
|---|---|
| Carbs | 51 g |
| Protein | 12 g |
| Fat | 18 g |
| Sodium | 180 mg |
| Fiber | 8 g |

*For Weight Gain*

| Calories | 820 kcal |
|---|---|
| Carbs | 102 g |
| Protein | 24 g |
| Fat | 36 g |
| Sodium | 360 mg |
| Fiber | 16 g |

**6-Ingredient Granola**

| Calories | 100 kcal |
|---|---|
| Carbs | 12 g |
| Protein | 2 g |
| Fat | 5 g |
| Sodium | 0 mg |
| Fiber | 2 g |

**Chia Pudding (plain)**

| Calories | 190 kcal |
|---|---|
| Carbs | 19 g |
| Protein | 7 g |
| Fat | 12 g |
| Sodium | 220 mg |
| Fiber | 13 g |
| Calcium | 510 mg |
| Vitamin E | 11 IU |
| Vitamin B12 | 2 mcg |

*For Weight Gain*

| Calories | 380 kcal |
|---|---|
| Carbs | 38 g |
| Protein | 14 g |
| Fat | 24 g |
| Sodium | 440 mg |
| Fiber | 26 g |
| Calcium | 1020 mg |
| Vitamin E | 22 IU |
| Vitamin B12 | 4 mcg |

**Tropical Chia Pudding**

| Calories | 350 kcal |
|---|---|
| Carbs | 33 g |
| Protein | 8 g |
| Fat | 24 g |
| Sodium | 220 mg |
| Fiber | 15 g |
| Vitamin A | 2068 IU |
| Vitamin C | 30 mg |
| Calcium | 529 mg |
| Vitamin E | 12 IU |
| Vitamin B12 | 2 mcg |

**Kiwi-Berry Chia Pudding**

| Calories | 300 kcal |
|---|---|
| Carbs | 33 g |
| Protein | 10 g |
| Fat | 18 g |
| Sodium | 230 mg |
| Fiber | 17 g |
| Vitamin C | 45 mg |
| Calcium | 559 mg |
| Vitamin B12 | 2 mcg |
| Vitamin E | 17 IU |
| Vitamin K | 25 mcg |

**Pressure Cooker Frittata**

| Calories | 112 kcal |
|---|---|
| Carbs | 2 g |
| Protein | 9 g |
| Fat | 6 g |
| Sodium | 290 mg |
| Fiber | 0 g |
| Vitamin E | 11 IU |
| Vitamin B12 | 2 mcg |

*For Weight Gain*

| Calories | 224 kcal |
|---|---|
| Carbs | 4 g |
| Protein | 18 g |
| Fat | 12 g |
| Sodium | 580 mg |
| Fiber | 1 g |
| Vitamin E | 22 IU |
| Vitamin B12 | 4 mcg |

**No-Sugar-Added Acai Bowl**

| Calories | 490 kcal |
|---|---|
| Carbs | 44 g |
| Protein | 10 g |
| Fat | 33 g |
| Sodium | 125 mg |
| Fiber | 10 g |
| Vitamin C | 26 mg |
| Calcium | 324 mg |
| Vitamin E | 9 IU |

# CHAPTER 7: SALADS, SOUPS, BOWLS, AND HANDHELDS

**Grilled Shrimp and Mango Salad with Cilantro-Lime Vinaigrette**

| Calories | 360 kcal |
|---|---|
| Carbs | 35 g |
| Protein | 9 g |
| Fat | 23 g |
| Sodium | 460 mg |
| Fiber | 5 g |
| Vitamin A | 5456 IU |
| Vitamin C | 69 mg |

**Anti-Inflammatory Salad with Honey-Lemon Vinaigrette**

| Calories | 327 kcal |
|---|---|
| Carbs | 25 g |
| Protein | 6 g |
| Fat | 26 g |
| Sodium | 26 mg |
| Fiber | 6 g |
| Vitamin A | 2597 IU |
| Vitamin C | 45 mg |
| Vitamin K | 189 mcg |

**Waldorf Kale Salad with Yogurt Dressing**

| Calories | 263 kcal |
|---|---|
| Carbs | 37 g |
| Protein | 9 g |
| Fat | 11 g |
| Sodium | 170 mg |
| Fiber | 6 g |
| Vitamin A | 1770 IU |
| Vitamin C | 27 mg |
| Vitamin K | 127 mcg |

**Southwest Chicken Soup**

| Calories | 305 kcal |
|---|---|
| Carbs | 36 g |
| Protein | 30 g |
| Fat | 5 g |
| Sodium | 780 mg |
| Fiber | 11 g |
| Vitamin C | 37 mg |

*For Weight Gain*

| Calories | 610 kcal |
|---|---|
| Carbs | 72 g |
| Protein | 60 g |
| Fat | 10 g |
| Sodium | 1560 mg |
| Fiber | 22 g |
| Vitamin C | 70 mg |

**Sweet Potato and Turkey Chili (without toppings)**

| Calories | 380 calories |
|---|---|
| Carbs | 50 g |
| Protein | 35 g |
| Fat | 4 g |
| Sodium | 740 mg |
| Fiber | 13 g |
| Vitamin A | 4269 IU |
| Vitamin C | 46 mg |
| Iron | 6 mg |
| Potassium | 374 mg |

*For Weight Gain*

| | |
|---|---|
| Calories | 760 calories |
| Carbs | 100 g |
| Protein | 70 g |
| Fat | 8 g |
| Sodium | 1480 mg |
| Fiber | 26 g |
| Vitamin A | 8538 IU |
| Vitamin C | 92 mg |
| Iron | 12 mg |
| Potassium | 748 mg |

### Lentil Chili

| | |
|---|---|
| Calories | 250 kcal |
| Carbs | 46 g |
| Protein | 12 g |
| Fat | 2.5 g |
| Sodium | 680 mg |
| Fiber | 12 g |
| Vitamin C | 39 mg |

*For Weight Gain*

| | |
|---|---|
| Calories | 500 kcal |
| Carbs | 92 g |
| Protein | 24 g |
| Fat | 5 g |
| Sodium | 1360 mg |
| Fiber | 24 g |
| Vitamin C | 78 mg |

### Chickpea-Lentil Curry

| | |
|---|---|
| Calories | 674 kcal |
| Carbs | 83 g |
| Protein | 21 g |
| Fat | 31 g |
| Sodium | 710 mg |
| Fiber | 14 g |
| Vitamin A | 6962 IU |
| Iron | 7 mg |
| Vitamin K | 42 mcg |

*For Weight Gain*

| | |
|---|---|
| Calories | 1348 kcal |
| Carbs | 166 g |
| Protein | 42 g |
| Fat | 62 g |
| Sodium | 1420 mg |
| Fiber | 28 g |
| Vitamin A | 13,924 IU |
| Iron | 14 mg |
| Vitamin K | 84 mcg |

### Shredded Salsa Chicken Burrito Bowls

| | |
|---|---|
| Calories | 340 kcal |
| Carbs | 40 g |
| Protein | 32 g |
| Fat | 5 g |

| | |
|---|---|
| Sodium | 810 mg |
| Fiber | 6 g |
| Vitamin A | 4472 IU |
| Vitamin K | 51 mcg |

*For Weight Gain*

| | |
|---|---|
| Calories | 680 kcal |
| Carbs | 80 g |
| Protein | 64 g |
| Fat | 10 g |
| Sodium | 1620 g |
| Fiber | 12 g |
| Vitamin A | 8944 IU |
| Vitamin K | 102 mcg |

### Ramen Bowls

| | |
|---|---|
| Calories | 450 kcal |
| Carbs | 34 g |
| Protein | 23 g |
| Fat | 24 g |
| Sodium | 1280 mg |
| Fiber | 4 g |
| Vitamin E | 11 IU |

*For Weight Gain*

| | |
|---|---|
| Calories | 900 kcal |
| Carbs | 68 g |
| Protein | 46 g |
| Fat | 48 g |
| Sodium | 2560 mg |
| Fiber | 8 g |
| Vitamin E | 22 IU |

### Vegan Buddha Bowls

| | |
|---|---|
| Calories | 637 kcal |
| Carbs | 85 g |
| Protein | 18 g |
| Fat | 28 g |
| Sodium | 450 mg |
| Fiber | 18 g |
| Vitamin A | 20,474 IU |
| Vitamin C | 27 mg |
| Potassium | 1153 mg |
| Magnesium | 130 mg |
| Vitamin K | 128 mcg |

### Buffalo Chicken Tacos with Ranch Dressing served with small flour tortillas

| | |
|---|---|
| Calories | 324 kcal |
| Carbs | 29 g |
| Protein | 22 g |
| Fat | 13 g |
| Sodium | 490 mg |
| Fiber | 2 g |
| Vitamin A | 4025 IU |

*For Weight Gain*

| | |
|---|---|
| Calories | 648 kcal |
| Carbs | 58 g |
| Protein | 44 g |
| Fat | 26 g |
| Sodium | 980 mg |
| Fiber | 4 g |
| Vitamin A | 8050 IU |

### Chicken Gyros served with 2 tablespoons tzatziki sauce

| | |
|---|---|
| Calories | 425 kcal |
| Carbs | 40 g |
| Protein | 35 g |
| Fat | 14 g |
| Sodium | 365 mg |
| Fiber | 5 g |

*For Weight Gain*

| | |
|---|---|
| Calories | 850 kcal |
| Carbs | 80 g |
| Protein | 70 g |
| Fat | 28 g |
| Sodium | 730 mg |
| Fiber | 10 g |

### Lentil Tacos

| | |
|---|---|
| Calories | 452 kcal |
| Carbs | 52 g |
| Protein | 17 g |
| Fat | 22 g |
| Sodium | 780 mg |
| Fiber | 17 g |
| Vitamin A | 3873 IU |
| Vitamin C | 22 mg |
| Iron | 7 mg |
| Potassium | 1109 mg |
| Vitamin K | 38 mcg |

*For Weight Gain*

| | |
|---|---|
| Calories | 904 kcal |
| Carbs | 104 g |
| Protein | 34 g |
| Fat | 44 g |
| Sodium | 1560 mg |
| Fiber | 34 g |
| Vitamin A | 7746 IU |
| Vitamin C | 44 mg |
| Iron | 14 mg |
| Potassium | 2218 mg |
| Vitamin K | 76 mcg |

### Chimichurri Mushroom Tacos

| | |
|---|---|
| Calories | 324 kcal |
| Carbs | 18 g |
| Protein | 3 g |

| | |
|---|---|
| Fat | 27 g |
| Sodium | 680 mg |
| Fiber | 4 g |
| Vitamin A | 1793 IU |
| Vitamin C | 26 mg |
| Vitamin K | 277 mcg |

*For Weight Gain*

| | |
|---|---|
| Calories | 648 kcal |
| Carbs | 36 g |
| Protein | 6 g |
| Fat | 54 g |
| Sodium | 1360 mg |
| Fiber | 8 g |
| Vitamin A | 3586 IU |
| Vitamin C | 52 mg |
| Vitamin K | 554 mcg |

### Fish Tacos with Pineapple-Mango Salsa served with small flour tortillas

| | |
|---|---|
| Calories | 330 kcal |
| Carbs | 34 g |
| Protein | 24 g |
| Fat | 11 g |
| Sodium | 1070 mg |
| Fiber | 3 g |
| Vitamin C | 49 mg |

*For Weight Gain*

| | |
|---|---|
| Calories | 660 kcal |
| Carbs | 68 g |
| Protein | 48 g |
| Fat | 22 g |
| Sodium | 2140 mg |
| Fiber | 6 g |
| Vitamin C | 98 mg |

# CHAPTER 8: MAINS

//////////////////////////////

### Tofu Parmesan

| | |
|---|---|
| Calories | 253 kcal |
| Carbs | 15 g |
| Protein | 20 g |
| Fat | 12 g |
| Sodium | 487 mg |
| Fiber | 5 g |

*For Weight Gain*

| | |
|---|---|
| Calories | 506 kcal |
| Carbs | 30 g |
| Protein | 40 g |
| Fat | 24 g |

| | |
|---|---|
| Sodium | 974 mg |
| Fiber | 10 g |

### Tofu Scramble

| | |
|---|---|
| Calories | 460 kcal |
| Carbs | 42 g |
| Protein | 20 g |
| Fat | 25 g |
| Sodium | 800 mg |
| Fiber | 8 g |
| Vitamin A | 1968 IU |
| Vitamin C | 120 mg |
| Vitamin B12 | 2 mcg |

*For Weight Gain*

| | |
|---|---|
| Calories | 920 kcal |
| Carbs | 84 g |
| Protein | 40 g |
| Fat | 50 g |
| Sodium | 1600 mg |
| Fiber | 16 g |
| Vitamin A | 3936 IU |
| Vitamin C | 240 mg |
| Vitamin B12 | 4 mcg |

### Spicy Pad Thai with Tofu

| | |
|---|---|
| Calories | 370 kcal |
| Carbs | 60 g |
| Protein | 16 g |
| Fat | 8 g |
| Sodium | 320 mg |
| Fiber | 7 g |
| Vitamin A | 3737 IU |
| Vitamin C | 55 mg |

*For Weight Gain*

| | |
|---|---|
| Calories | 740 kcal |
| Carbs | 120 g |
| Protein | 32 g |
| Fat | 16 g |
| Sodium | 640 mg |
| Fiber | 14 g |
| Vitamin A | 7474 IU |
| Vitamin C | 110 mg |

### Tempeh Bolognese served without pasta or vegetables

| | |
|---|---|
| Calories | 234 kcal |
| Carbs | 25 g |
| Protein | 15 g |
| Fat | 8 g |
| Sodium | 522 mg |
| Fiber | 10 g |
| Vitamin C | 19 mg |

*For Weight Gain*

| | |
|---|---|
| Calories | 468 kcal |
| Carbs | 50 g |
| Protein | 30 g |
| Fat | 16 g |
| Sodium | 1044 mg |
| Fiber | 20 g |
| Vitamin C | 38 mg |

### Simple Baked Salmon

| | |
|---|---|
| Calories | 308 kcal |
| Carbs | 19 g |
| Protein | 32 g |
| Fat | 11 g |
| Sodium | 279 mg |
| Fiber | 1 g |
| Potassium | 759 mg |
| Vitamin B12 | 4.6 mcg |

*For Weight Gain*

| | |
|---|---|
| Calories | 616 kcal |
| Carbs | 38 g |
| Protein | 64 g |
| Fat | 22 g |
| Sodium | 558 mg |
| Fiber | 2 g |
| Potassium | 1518 mg |
| Vitamin B12 | 9.2 mcg |

### One-Pan Salmon and Roasted Vegetables

| | |
|---|---|
| Calories | 450 kcal |
| Carbs | 15 g |
| Protein | 46 g |
| Fat | 21 g |
| Sodium | 350 mg |
| Fiber | 1 g |
| Vitamin C | 27 mg |
| Vitamin B12 | 7 mcg |

*For Weight Gain*

| | |
|---|---|
| Calories | 900 kcal |
| Carbs | 30 g |
| Protein | 92 g |
| Fat | 42 g |
| Sodium | 700 kcal |
| Fiber | 2 g |
| Vitamin C | 54 mg |
| Vitamin B12 | 14 mcg |

### Whole-Grain Pesto Fusilli with Scallops served with 1 tablespoon grated parmesan cheese

| | |
|---|---|
| Calories | 436 kcal |
| Carbs | 51 g |

| | |
|---|---|
| Protein | 28 g |
| Fat | 15 g |
| Sodium | 707 mg |
| Fiber | 7 g |
| Vitamin A | 1634 IU |
| Vitamin C | 49 mg |
| Magnesium | 133 mg |
| Vitamin K | 48 mcg |

*For Weight Gain*

| | |
|---|---|
| Calories | 872 kcal |
| Carbs | 102 g |
| Protein | 56 g |
| Fat | 30 g |
| Sodium | 1414 mg |
| Fiber | 14 g |
| Vitamin A | 3268 IU |
| Vitamin C | 98 mg |
| Magnesium | 266 mg |
| Vitamin K | 96 mcg |

### Shrimp and Broccoli Stir-Fry

| | |
|---|---|
| Calories | 410 kcal |
| Carbs | 59 g |
| Protein | 22 g |
| Fat | 10 g |
| Sodium | 1380 mg |
| Fiber | 4 g |
| Vitamin C | 41 mg |
| Vitamin K | 48 mcg |

*For Weight Gain*

| | |
|---|---|
| Calories | 820 kcal |
| Carbs | 118 g |
| Protein | 44 g |
| Fat | 20 g |
| Sodium | 2760 mg |
| Fiber | 8 g |
| Vitamin C | 82 mg |
| Vitamin K | 96 mcg |

### Turkey Bolognese

| | |
|---|---|
| Calories | 210 kcal |
| Carbs | 15 g |
| Protein | 30 g |
| Fat | 4 g |
| Sodium | 410 mg |
| Fiber | 4 g |
| Vitamin C | 31 mg |
| Vitamin K | 24 mcg |

*For Weight Gain*

| | |
|---|---|
| Calories | 420 kcal |
| Carbs | 30 g |
| Protein | 60 g |
| Fat | 8 g |
| Sodium | 820 mg |

| | |
|---|---|
| Fiber | 8 g |
| Vitamin C | 62 mg |
| Vitamin K | 48 mcg |

### Turkey Burgers

| | |
|---|---|
| Calories | 180 kcal |
| Carbs | 2 g |
| Protein | 27 g |
| Fat | 6 g |
| Sodium | 125 mg |
| Fiber | 0 g |

*For Weight Gain*

| | |
|---|---|
| Calories | 360 kcal |
| Carbs | 4 g |
| Protein | 54 g |
| Fat | 12 g |
| Sodium | 250 mg |
| Fiber | 0 g |

### Slow or Instant Turkey Meatballs

| | |
|---|---|
| Calories | 230 kcal |
| Carbs | 14 g |
| Protein | 27 g |
| Fat | 6 g |
| Sodium | 640 mg |
| Fiber | 4 g |
| Vitamin K | 35 mcg |

*For Weight Gain*

| | |
|---|---|
| Calories | 460 kcal |
| Carbs | 28 g |
| Protein | 54 g |
| Fat | 12 g |
| Sodium | 1280 mg |
| Fiber | 8 g |
| Vitamin K | 70 mcg |

### Chicken Meatballs served with The Primal Kitchen alfredo sauce

| | |
|---|---|
| Calories | 260 kcal |
| Carbs | 8 g |
| Protein | 32 g |
| Fat | 11 g |
| Sodium | 890 mg |
| Fiber | 1 g |

*For Weight Gain*

| | |
|---|---|
| Calories | 520 kcal |
| Carbs | 16 g |
| Protein | 64 g |
| Fat | 22 g |
| Sodium | 1780 mg |
| Fiber | 2 g |

## Shredded Buffalo Chicken

| | |
|---|---|
| Calories | 185 kcal |
| Carbs | 10 g |
| Protein | 26 g |
| Fat | 4 g |
| Sodium | 290 mg |
| Fiber | 0 g |

*For Weight Gain*

| | |
|---|---|
| Calories | 370 kcal |
| Carbs | 20 g |
| Protein | 52 g |
| Fat | 8 g |
| Sodium | 580 mg |
| Fiber | 0 g |

## Bruschetta Chicken

| | |
|---|---|
| Calories | 280 kcal |
| Carbs | 12 g |
| Protein | 42 g |
| Fat | 7 g |
| Sodium | 190 mg |
| Fiber | 2 g |

*For Weight Gain*

| | |
|---|---|
| Calories | 560 kcal |
| Carbs | 24 g |
| Protein | 84 g |
| Fat | 14 g |
| Sodium | 380 mg |
| Fiber | 4 g |

## Mediterranean Chicken

| | |
|---|---|
| Calories | 343 kcal |
| Carbs | 1 g |
| Protein | 38 g |
| Fat | 20 g |
| Sodium | 65 mg |
| Fiber | 0 g |

*For Weight Gain*

| | |
|---|---|
| Calories | 686 kcal |
| Carbs | 2 g |
| Protein | 76 g |
| Fat | 40 g |
| Sodium | 130 g |
| Fiber | 0 g |

## Thai Peanut Chicken

| | |
|---|---|
| Calories | 464 kcal |
| Carbs | 36 g |
| Protein | 34 g |
| Fat | 19 g |
| Sodium | 610 mg |
| Fiber | 4 g |

*For Weight Gain*

| | |
|---|---|
| Calories | 928 kcal |
| Carbs | 72 g |
| Protein | 68 g |
| Fat | 38 g |
| Sodium | 1220 mg |
| Fiber | 8 g |

## Buffalo Chicken Pizza

| | |
|---|---|
| Calories | 344 kcal |
| Carbs | 38 g |
| Protein | 26 g |
| Fat | 12 g |
| Sodium | 658 mg |
| Fiber | 6 g |

## Pesto Baked Chicken with 1 teaspoon basil pesto

| | |
|---|---|
| Calories | 257 kcal |
| Carbs | 3.5 g |
| Protein | 42 g |
| Fat | 7.5 g |
| Sodium | 200 mg |
| Fiber | 1 g |

*For Weight Gain*

| | |
|---|---|
| Calories | 514 kcal |
| Carbs | 7 g |
| Protein | 84 g |
| Fat | 15 g |
| Sodium | 400 mg |
| Fiber | 2 g |

## Mexican-Inspired Chicken Casserole

| | |
|---|---|
| Calories | 426 kcal |
| Carbs | 45 g |
| Protein | 36 g |
| Fat | 12 g |
| Sodium | 770 mg |
| Fiber | 9 g |
| Vitamin C | 30 mg |
| Calcium | 285 mg |
| Vitamin K | 17 mcg |

*For Weight Gain*

| | |
|---|---|
| Calories | 852 kcal |
| Carbs | 90 g |
| Protein | 72 g |
| Fat | 24 g |
| Sodium | 1540 mg |
| Fiber | 18 g |
| Vitamin C | 60 mg |
| Calcium | 570 mg |
| Vitamin K | 34 mcg |

## Honey-Garlic Chicken

| | |
|---|---|
| Calories | 340 kcal |
| Carbs | 45 g |
| Protein | 31 g |
| Fat | 4 g |
| Sodium | 250 mg |
| Fiber | 1 g |

*For Weight Gain*

| | |
|---|---|
| Calories | 680 kcal |
| Carbs | 90 g |
| Protein | 62 g |
| Fat | 8 g |
| Sodium | 500 mg |
| Fiber | 2 g |

## Almond-Crusted Chicken with Baked Potato Chips

| | |
|---|---|
| Calories | 490 kcal |
| Carbs | 40 g |
| Protein | 38 g |
| Fat | 21 g |
| Sodium | 705 mg |
| Fiber | 5 g |

*For Weight Gain*

| | |
|---|---|
| Calories | 980 kcal |
| Carbs | 80 g |
| Protein | 76 g |
| Fat | 42 g |
| Sodium | 1410 mg |
| Fiber | 10 g |

## Lemon-Garlic Marinated Chicken

| | |
|---|---|
| Calories | 250 kcal |
| Carbs | 2 g |
| Protein | 39 g |
| Fat | 9 g |
| Sodium | 190 mg |
| Fiber | 1 g |

*For Weight Gain*

| | |
|---|---|
| Calories | 500 kcal |
| Carbs | 4 g |
| Protein | 78 g |
| Fat | 18 g |
| Sodium | 380 mg |
| Fiber | 2 g |

## Barbecue Chicken with Baked Sweet Potatoes and Steamed Collard Greens

| | |
|---|---|
| Calories | 472 kcal |
| Carbs | 31 g |
| Protein | 42 g |

| | |
|---|---|
| Fat | 21 g |
| Sodium | 367 mg |
| Fiber | 5 g |
| Vitamin A | 19,094 IU |
| Vitamin K | 88 mcg |

*For Weight Gain*

| | |
|---|---|
| Calories | 944 kcal |
| Carbs | 62 g |
| Protein | 84 g |
| Fat | 42 g |
| Sodium | 734 mg |
| Fiber | 10 g |
| Vitamin A | 38,188 IU |
| Vitamin K | 175 mcg |

## One-Pan Chicken and Veggie Dinner

| | |
|---|---|
| Calories | 364 kcals |
| Carbs | 42 g |
| Protein | 31 g |
| Fat | 9 g |
| Sodium | 170 mg |
| Fiber | 6 g |
| Potassium | 1111 mg |
| Vitamin C | 65 mg |
| Vitamin K | 48 mcg |

*For Weight Gain*

| | |
|---|---|
| Calories | 728 kcal |
| Carbs | 84 g |
| Protein | 62 g |
| Fat | 18 g |
| Sodium | 340 mg |
| Fiber | 12 g |
| Potassium | **2222 mg** |
| Vitamin C | 130 mg |
| Vitamin K | 96 mcg |

# CHAPTER 9: PERFORMANCE SNACKS AND SWEET TREATS

## Post-Workout Recovery Bites made with honey

| | |
|---|---|
| Calories | 93 kcal |
| Carbs | 10 g |
| Protein | 4 g |
| Fat | 4 g |

| Sodium | 25 mg |
|---|---|
| Fiber | 2 g |

**Homemade Sports Drinks**

| Calories | 122 kcal |
|---|---|
| Carbs | 29 g |
| Protein | 2 g |
| Fat | 0 g |
| Sodium | 290–580 mg |
| Fiber | 0 g |
| Vitamin C | 121 mg |
| Potassium | 700 mg |

**3-Ingredient Energy Bars**

| Calories | 136 kcal |
|---|---|
| Carbs | 16 g |
| Protein | 3 g |
| Fat | 7 g |
| Sodium | 25 mg |
| Fiber | 3 g |

**Endurance Trail Mix made with Cascadian Farm Purely O's cereal**

| Calories | 257 kcal |
|---|---|
| Carbs | 14 g |
| Protein | 9 g |
| Fat | 20 g |
| Sodium | 100 mg |
| Fiber | 3 g |
| Magnesium | 120 mg |

**Parmesan-Roasted Edamame**

| Calories | 155 kcal |
|---|---|
| Carbs | 8 g |
| Protein | 11 g |
| Fat | 9 g |
| Sodium | 265 mg |
| Fiber | 4 g |

**Roasted Chickpeas**

| Calories | 160 kcal |
|---|---|
| Carbs | 20 g |
| Protein | 6 g |
| Fat | 7 g |
| Sodium | 180 mg |
| Fiber | 5 g |

**Cashew Queso**

| Calories | 150 kcal |
|---|---|
| Carbs | 12 g |
| Protein | 8 g |

| Fat | 8 g |
|---|---|
| Sodium | 214 mg |
| Fiber | 3 g |
| Vitamin B12 | 4 mcg |

**Avocado Toast with Hard-Boiled Eggs**

| Calories | 320 kcal |
|---|---|
| Carbs | 24 g |
| Protein | 19 g |
| Fat | 17 g |
| Sodium | 240 mg |
| Fiber | 4 g |

**Almond Zucchini Muffins**

| Calories | 140 kcal |
|---|---|
| Carbs | 10 g |
| Protein | 5 g |
| Fat | 9 g |
| Sodium | 270 mg |
| Fiber | 2 g |

**Blueberry Muffins**

| Calories | 200 kcal |
|---|---|
| Carbs | 29 g |
| Protein | 5 g |
| Fat | 7 g |
| Sodium | 115 mg |
| Fiber | 5 g |

**Chocolate Chip Banana Bread**

| Calories | 233 kcal |
|---|---|
| Carbs | 21 g |
| Protein | 7 g |
| Fat | 15 g |
| Sodium | 163 mg |
| Fiber | 4 g |
| Iron | 3 mg |

**Almond Flour Chocolate Chip Cookies**

| Calories | 90 kcal |
|---|---|
| Carbs | 8 g |
| Protein | 1 g |
| Fat | 6 g |
| Sodium | 60 mg |
| Fiber | 1 g |

**Raw Cookie Dough**

| Calories | 164 kcal |
|---|---|
| Carbs | 13 g |
| Protein | 4 g |
| Fat | 11 g |

| Sodium | 75 mg |
|---|---|
| Fiber | 2 g |

**No-Bake Brownies**

| Calories | 237 kcal |
|---|---|
| Carbs | 27 g |
| Protein | 4 g |
| Fat | 14 g |
| Sodium | 15 mg |
| Fiber | 5 g |

**Vegan Peanut Butter Cookies**

| Calories | 145 kcal |
|---|---|
| Carbs | 11 g |
| Protein | 5 g |
| Fat | 11 g |
| Sodium | 80 mg |
| Fiber | 2 g |

**Slow Cooker Peach-Apple Crisp**

| Calories | 277 kcal |
|---|---|
| Carbs | 46 g |
| Protein | 4 g |
| Fat | 10 g |
| Sodium | 2 mg |
| Fiber | 6 g |

**Dark Chocolate Nut Clusters with ¼ cup nuts for topping**

| Calories | 170 kcal |
|---|---|
| Carbs | 11 g |
| Protein | 3 g |
| Fat | 13 g |
| Sodium | 22 mg |
| Fiber | 3 g |

**Avocado Mousse**

| Calories | 218 kcal |
|---|---|
| Carbs | 26 g |
| Protein | 3 g |
| Fat | 13 g |
| Sodium | 15 mg |
| Fiber | 4 g |

**Avocado Mousse made with peanut butter**

| Calories | 260 kcal |
|---|---|
| Carbs | 27 g |
| Protein | 4 g |
| Fat | 16 g |
| Sodium | 35 mg |
| Fiber | 5 g |

**Frozen Berry Yogurt Bites**

| Calories | 50 kcal |
|---|---|
| Carbs | 11 g |
| Protein | 2 g |
| Fat | 0 g |
| Sodium | 5 mg |
| Fiber | 2 g |

**Blueberry-Lemon Tarts**

| Calories | 141 kcal |
|---|---|
| Carbs | 13 g |
| Protein | 4 g |
| Fat | 9 g |
| Sodium | 9 mg |
| Fiber | 2 g |

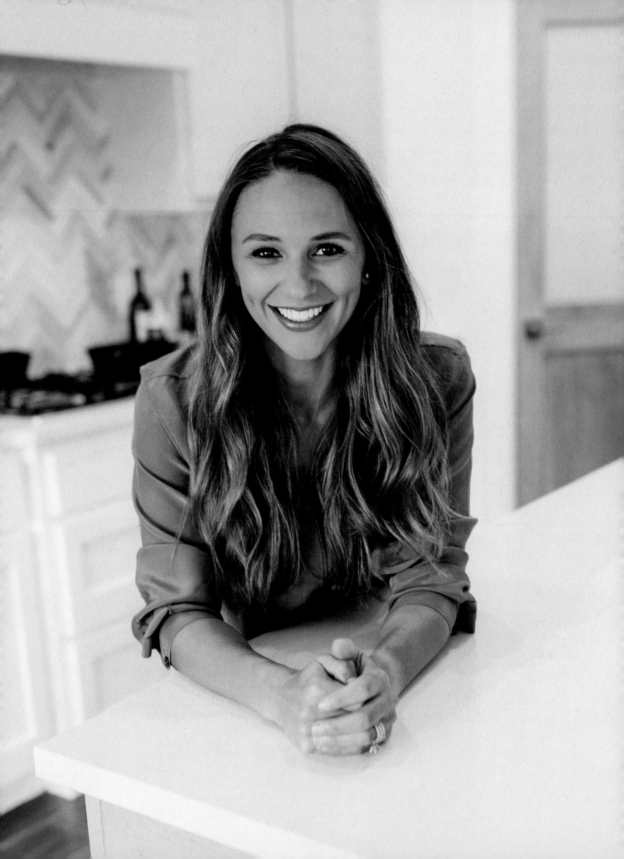

# ACKNOWLEDGMENTS

## I WOULD LIKE TO THANK . . .

My husband, Cody. I feel overwhelmed with gratitude for the love and support you constantly provide. Thank you for believing in me; for always being there whenever I need an editor, a taste tester, advice, or words of encouragement. None of this would have been possible without you.

My parents. Mom, for the countless hours you spent cooking from scratch, for teaching us three kids the importance of family dinners and trying new foods, and for being the first to teach me how to cook. And most importantly, for being the most patient and loving person I know. Dad, for being my greatest mentor and inspiration and for shaping me into the person I am today. I aspire to be more like you every single day.

Kandyce and Jermelle Cudjo, for your unrivaled friendship and generosity. Thank you for allowing me to turn your home into a cookbook test kitchen, for taste testing nearly every recipe in this book, for being my number one fans from day one, and for being the most kindhearted clients turned best friends.

My agent, Amy Levenson, for helping me navigate through this experience I knew so little about just one year ago.

My editor, Jessica Easto, and designer, Morgan Krehbiel, as well as the entire team at Agate Publishing. Thank you for making my dream a reality, for understanding the importance of this book, and for turning it into something even more incredible than I could have imagined.

Katie Hass of kgc photography, Casey Haley, Liz Jirschele, and Hayley Dolson for the beautiful work you did in making my recipes come to life. Katie, you are an unbelievably talented photographer and an even better friend. Thank you for investing so much of your time into these photos.

All of my clients, past and current, who have truly been the inspiration for so many of the recipes throughout this cookbook. And finally, to the thousands of you who have been following and supporting Eleat Sports Nutrition over the years. I am so grateful for the support you provide, and I hope you enjoy this book as much as I enjoyed creating it.

# SIMPLE MEASUREMENT CONVERSION GUIDE

## WEIGHT

1 kilogram (kg) = 2.2 pounds (lb)

1 pound = 16 ounces = 453 grams

8 ounces = 227 grams

4 ounces = 113 grams

1 ounce = 28 grams

## MEASUREMENTS

1 cup = 8 fluid ounces = 240 milliliters = 16 tablespoons

¾ cup = 6 fluid ounces = 177 milliliters = 12 tablespoons

½ cup = 4 fluid ounces = 118 milliliters = 8 tablespoons

¼ cup = 2 fluid ounces = 59 milliliters = 4 tablespoons

1 tablespoon = 3 teaspoons

## TEMPERATURE

350°F = 180°C

375°F = 190°C

400°F = 200°C

425°F = 220° C

A "pinch" of salt or black pepper = $\frac{1}{16}$ teaspoon

Fresh herbs to dried herbs = 3:1 ratio;
use 1 teaspoon dried for 1 tablespoon (3 teaspoons) fresh

# INDEX

# ABOUT THE AUTHOR

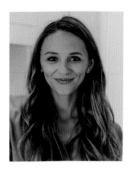 **ANGIE ASCHE** is a nationally recognized food and nutrition expert, a board-certified specialist in sports dietetics, and a certified exercise physiologist. Her professional experience began after obtaining a dual Bachelor of Science degree in Dietetics and Exercise Science from the University of Nebraska–Lincoln. She went on to complete her dietetic internship and Master of Science in Nutrition and Physical Performance at Saint Louis University. She realized early on that her passion was sports nutrition and studying the profound impact nutrition can have on athletic performance, which led her to launch her private practice in 2014.

Since founding Eleat Sports Nutrition, Angie has worked with hundreds of high school, college, and professional athletes nationwide, including those in MLB, NHL, and NFL. Angie has also worked as the nutrition consultant to the University of Nebraska–Lincoln volleyball team. While she works with competitive athletes in a variety of sports, her primary clientele is baseball players. Her husband, Cody Asche, is a professional baseball player and has played in MLB for the Philadelphia Phillies and Chicago White Sox, so Angie understands on both a professional and a personal level the difficulties that athletes face when it comes to nutrition.

Angie currently resides in Nebraska and travels across the country to consult with athletes. In her spare time, she enjoys running with her dog, racing in triathlons, and traveling with her husband. She can be found at eleatnutrition.com and on Instagram @eleatnutrition.